MASSACHUSETTS GENERAL HOSPITAL

NURSING *at* TWO HUNDRED

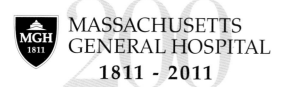

MASSACHUSETTS GENERAL HOSPITAL
1811 - 2011

Massachusetts General Hospital Department of Nursing
55 Fruit Street, Bulfinch 230
Boston, MA 02114

Published by Jeanette Ives Erickson, RN, MS, FAAN
Edited by Georgia W. Peirce with Marianne Ditomassi, RN, MSN, MBA
Designed by Georgia W. Peirce
Printed by Kirkwood Printing

Manufactured in the United States of America

Library of Congress Control Number: 2011924104

ISBN 0-6154-4023-1

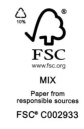

FSC
www.fsc.org
MIX
Paper from
responsible sources
FSC® C002933

MASSACHUSETTS GENERAL HOSPITAL

Nursing *at* Two Hundred

SPECIAL THANKS

This book was made possible in large part through the enthusiasm and efforts of a small group of dedicated volunteers. Throughout the course of more than a year, they spent countless hours rediscovering, researching and writing about pieces of MGH nursing history long forgotten. Thank you to the members of the *MGH Nursing at Two Hundred* Book Committee:

Patricia Austen, RN

Patricia Beckles, RN

Gino Chisari, RN

Ann Collins, RN

Marianne Ditomassi, RN

Barbara Dunderdale, RN

Susan Fisher, RN

Mary Larkin, RN

Michelle Marcella

Roberta Nemeskal, RN

Linda Orrell, RN

Georgia Peirce

Hannah Potter

Susan Sabia

Martha Stone

ACKNOWLEDGEMENTS

The MGH Department of Nursing would like to acknowledge the MGH Nurses' Alumnae Association, which has preserved much of the MGH Nursing history that might otherwise have been lost through the years; Helen Sherwin, who initially organized the MGH School of Nursing Archives; Sara E. Parsons, who wrote *The History of the Massachusetts General Hospital Training School for Nurses*; Sylvia Perkins, author of *A Centennial Review: the Massachusetts General Hospital School of Nursing 1873-1973*; Patient Care Services Communication interns Milourdes "Mimi" Augustin, Sarah Otterstetter and Alexandra Sliwkowski, who brought fresh eyes, energy and ideas to the project; Georgia Peirce and Marianne Ditomassi for their leadership and vision, which guided the project from the outset. Thanks also go to the MGH Photography Department and the MGH Office of Public Affairs; director emeritus Edward Coakley, The Center for Innovations in Care Delivery; Maureen Greenberg, Patient Care Services Administration; Maureen Larkin, MGH Human Resources; Jeff Mifflin, MGH Archives and Special Collections; Bob Riseman, Kirkwood Printing; and Jane Winton, Prints Department, Boston Public Library.

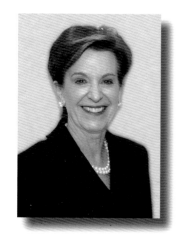

The MGH bicentennial offers a rare opportunity to celebrate our history — to reflect upon the various milestones and people who brought us to where we are today.

As we begin to explore the past two centuries of nursing at the Massachusetts General Hospital, we are literally looking at the earliest days of nursing in America. We see the emergence of the "trained" nurse and the development of nursing practice. We watch as that practice advances decade after decade. And we come to recognize that many of those who helped to establish and advance the profession of nursing in our country and throughout the world were directly influenced by their experiences at MGH.

We also see the striking emergence of many familiar themes: a relentless commitment to providing the best available care to those in need; advancing that care through life-long learning; attaining and sharing knowledge broadly; contributing to the profession as a whole; and serving our country and our neighbors, near and far.

The pages that follow feature recollections from MGH nurses of the mid- and late 1800s and those more recent, photographs long forgotten and others quite familiar. While it is impossible to include every story, photograph, artifact or even milestone, *MGH Nursing at Two Hundred* provides a compelling glimpse of just how far nursing has progressed in 200 years.

It also becomes clear that ours is a legacy of leadership. It is my privilege to work among those who are helping to write the next chapter.

With admiration,

Jeanette Ives Erickson

Jeanette Ives Erickson, RN, MS, FAAN
Senior Vice President for Patient Care and Chief Nurse

Dedicated to the many MGH nurses

who throughout the past 200 years

contributed to a legacy of

excellence in patient care ... and to those

with whom that is now entrusted.

...n, Thomas Aldridge, Ja...

onathan Harris, James Mann, Timothy Childs, Daniel

...ll, Andrew Craigie, John Warren, Richard Sullivan, and

...of the Corporation herein after created, according to the bye La...

...e name of The Massachusetts General Hospital, a...

...hem devised, altered, and renewed at their pleasure. ⸺

...d, That the said Corporation, may take and receive, hold, pu...

...itution, any grants, and devises of lands and tenements, in f...

...erty, to be used and improved for the erection, support, and m...

...e of said Corporation, from its real and personal estate ...

⸺

...ted, That it shall be in the power of the Legislature of this C...

...oduce into the said Hospital all such lunatick and sick,...

...t and medical, and other necessary aid and assistance, at the ...

...for them therein suitable apartments, bed-clothing, board, an...

...the sole charge of the funds of the Corporation. Provided t...

...f officers appointed by them for that purpose, shall, at no on...

...further number of the state's poor. ⸺

...cted, That in consideration of the obligation aforesaid imposed...

...e House, with all the lands under and appurtenant to the sa...

On February 25, 1811, the Massachusetts Legislature granted a charter to establish the Massachusetts General Hospital.

...h sale shall be made, the said Corporation shall give bo...

In 1810, health care in Boston was by all measures rudimentary.
There was no organized system of health care
and no general hospital in New England.
Those who could afford care were treated in their homes.
"Nurses" were virtually untrained; there was
no formalized school of nursing in America.
And the poor were cared for in an almshouse or "poor house."

It was becoming clear that Boston needed a middle ground
between expensive private medical care and the almshouse.

On March 8, 1810, Reverend John Bartlett, chaplain of the city's almshouse that provided care to Boston's poor, met with notable Boston physicians John Collins Warren and James Jackson. They discussed the possibility of establishing a hospital in Boston — a facility that could offer health care to the poor and most vulnerable and provide a place for medical training. The doctors were charged with calling upon the people of Boston to raise funds for this unprecedented and noble vision. A letter dated the following day stated their intent to form a committee "on the expediency of establishing a General Hospital for the reception of the sick, lunatics and pregnant women, who may seek such an asylum."

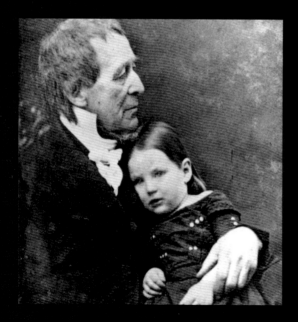

Dr. James Jackson with his granddaughter

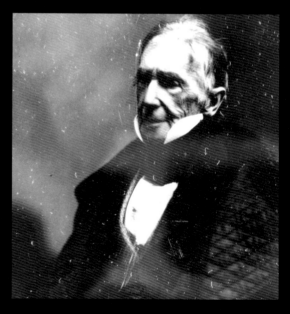

Dr. John Collins Warren

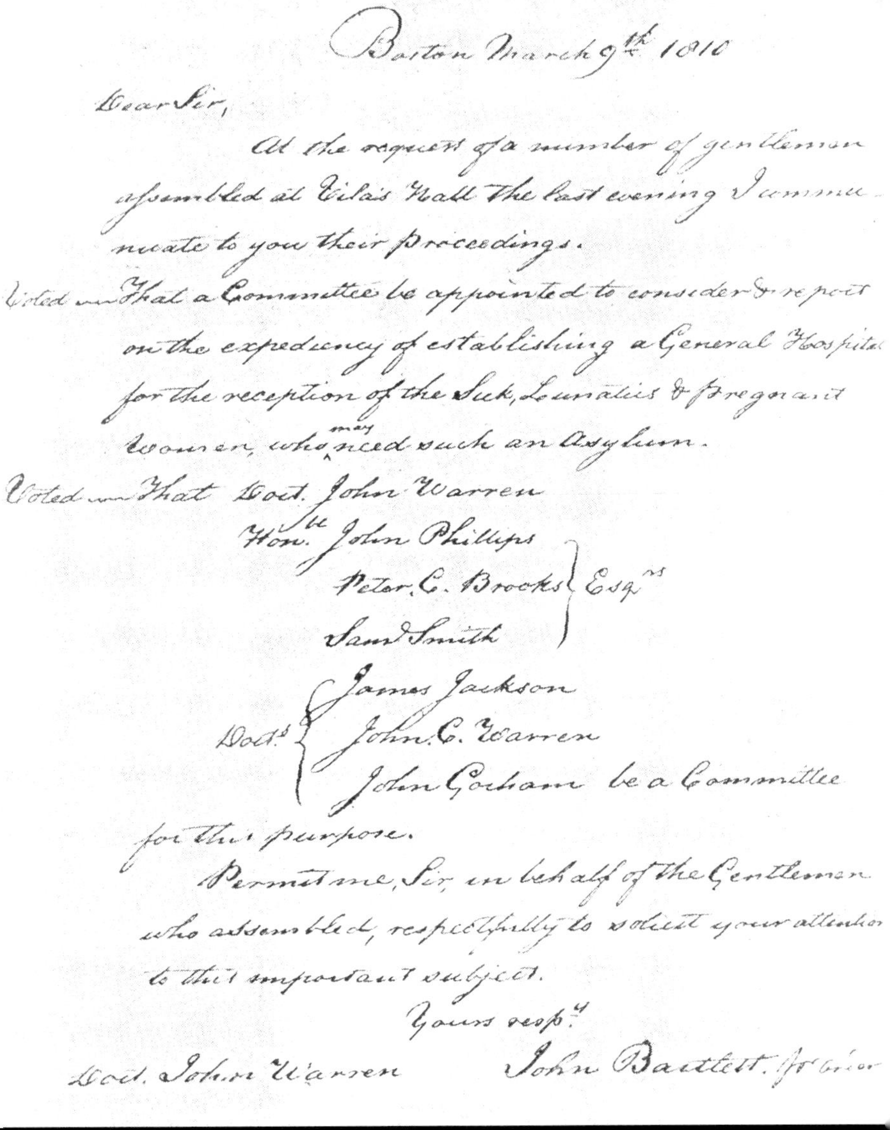

Boston March 9th 1810

Dear Sir,

At the request of a number of gentlemen assembled at Vila's Hall the last evening I communicate to you their proceedings.

Voted — That a Committee be appointed to consider & report on the expediency of establishing a General Hospital for the reception of the Sick, Lunatics & Pregnant women, who may need such an Asylum.

Voted — That Doct. John Warren
Hon.ble John Phillips
Peter C. Brooks
Saml Smith } Esqrs
Docts { James Jackson
John C. Warren
John Gorham } be a Committee for this purpose.

Permit me, Sir, in behalf of the Gentlemen who assembled, respectfully to solicit your attention to this important subject.

Yours respy

John Bartlett. for Com

Doct. John Warren

A letter dated March 9, 1810, and signed by Dr. John Warren, cofounder of Harvard Medical School, and Rev. John Bartlett, chaplain of the city's almshouse, proposed that a committee be established to report on the expediency of establishing a general hospital. The members listed were Dr. John Warren; the Hon. John Phillips; Attys. Peter C. Brooks and Samuel Smith; and Drs. James Jackson, John C. Warren and John Gorham

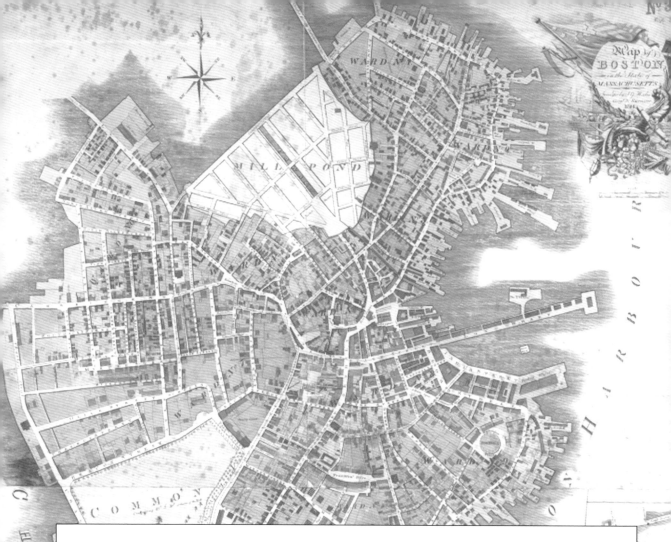

In general, the early 1800s were difficult years to ask Bostonians for donations for the proposed hospital. In 1807, U.S. President Thomas Jefferson found himself caught in a trade battle between Britain and France and declared an embargo, closing all American ports to foreign trade. This severely affected the trade-based New England economy, and Boston suffered. The War of 1812 made fund raising even more difficult, resulting in a 10-year gap between the signing of the MGH charter and the eventual opening of the hospital.

Map reproduction courtesy of the Norman B. Leventhal Map Center at the Boston Public Library

On August 20, 1810, Jackson and Warren distributed a letter to friends, colleagues and prominent citizens of Boston articulating the need for a general hospital and requesting financial support for this ambitious undertaking. Their plea for support described how the poor and disenfranchised could find care, comfort and hope in a hospital. In post-Colonial Boston, such individuals had few places to turn when sick or injured.

While the language of the MGH "circular letter" clearly speaks from another era, the sentiment and spirit in the letter's passages are noteworthy for their passion, their boldness and their vision — and their appreciation of nursing. "When in distress every man becomes our neighbor," the document proclaimed.

"It has appeared very desirable to a number of respectable gentlemen, that a hospital for the reception of ... sick persons should be established in this town. ... When in distress, every man becomes our neighbour."

"In this wretched situation the sick man is destitute of all those common conveniences, without which most of us would consider it impossible to live, even in health. Wholesome food and sufficient fuel are wanting; and his own sufferings are aggravated by the cries of hungry children. Above all, he suffers from the want of that first requisite in sickness, a kind and skillful nurse."

"In a well regulated hospital they would find a comfortable lodging in a duly attempered atmosphere; would receive the food best suited to their various conditions; and would be attended by kind and discreet nurses, under the direction of a physician. In such a situation the poor man's chance for relief would be equal perhaps to that of the most affluent, when affected with the same disease."

Bostonians were inspired to heed the call. As encouragement and funds grew, the idea of a general hospital in Boston began to take shape. On February 25, 1811, the Massachusetts Legislature granted a charter to establish the Massachusetts General Hospital. Finally, on July 4, 1818, the cornerstone of the Bulfinch Building was laid.

The Bulfinch Building opened in 1821 as the original Massachusetts General Hospital structure. Located on a bank of the Charles River, it was accessible by land and sea. This photo, taken in the late 1850s, shows evidence of early hospital expansion. To the right is the old Harvard Medical School; to the far left, "the Brick" or "Foul Ward," was constructed to serve as the hospital's isolation ward. The hospital's first student nurses were assigned to the Brick, which in 1874 was converted into their residence.

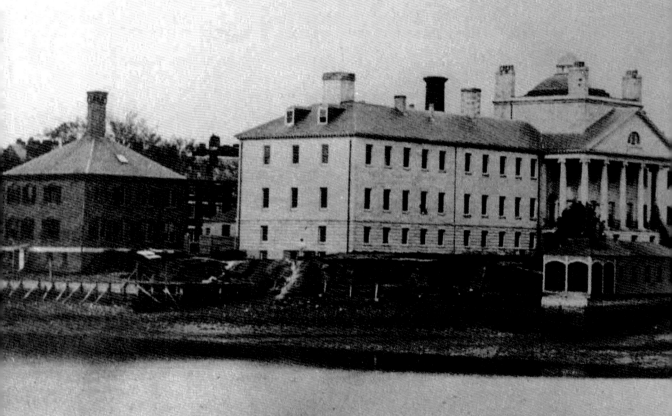

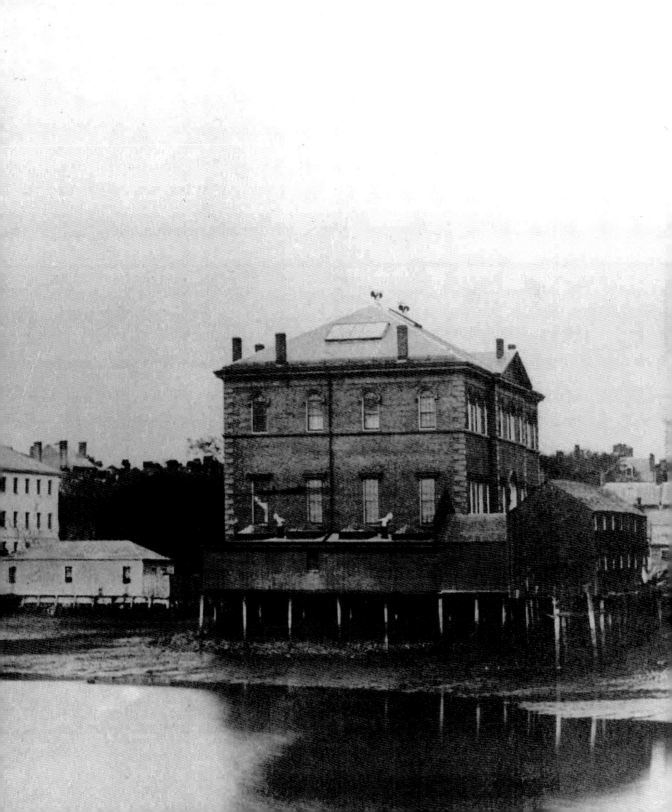

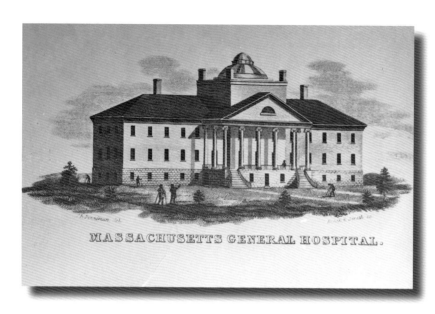

MASSACHUSETTS GENERAL HOSPITAL.

On September 3, 1821, the Massachusetts General Hospital admitted its first patient, a 30-year-old saddler, according to Volume I of the Massachusetts General Hospital Medical Records (housed in the MGH Archives and Special Collections).

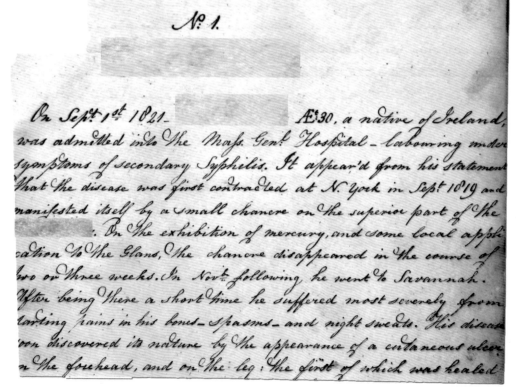

No 1.

On Sept. 1st 1821 — Æt 30, a native of Ireland, was admitted into the Mass. Genl. Hospital — labouring under symptoms of secondary Syphilis. It appear'd from his statement that the disease was first contracted at N. York in Sept. 1819 and manifested itself by a small chancre on the superior part of the ___. On the exhibition of mercury, and some local appli-cation to the Glans, the chancre disappeared in the course of two or three weeks. In Novr. following, he went to Savannah. After being there a short time he suffered most severely from darting pains in his bones — Spasms — and night sweats. His disease soon discovered its nature by the appearance of a cutaneous ulcer on the forehead, and on the leg: the first of which was healed

Please note that the patient's name was removed from the above document to comply with current privacy regulations.

The earliest known documentation of a nurse being hired at the MGH can be found in the minutes of the hospital's Visiting Committee dated October 18, 1821. It is believed that the nurse was the wife of the MGH's first patient. It is possible she sought work when her husband could not pay his bill of $3 per week.

"Oct. 18th, 1821. The Committee met. Mrs. [name] wife of ... one of the patients came to the Hospital ... having been engaged by the Superintendent as a Nurse at seven dollars per month."

Please note that the patient's name was removed from the above documentation to comply with current privacy regulations.

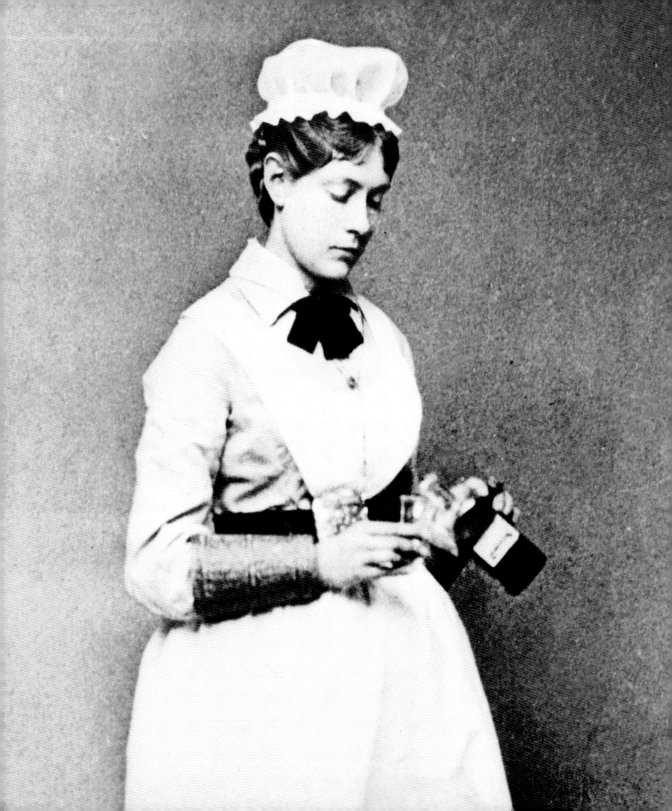

"How high are the duties of a nurse; and how justly they entitle one, who performs them skillfully and faithfully and kindly, to the love and respect of mankind."

— James Jackson, MD, MGH Cofounder

"We offer to you then ... kind nurses, whose only duty and occupation it is to watch and provide for the sick; proper and nourishing food; rest and tranquility; ... [and] physicians, nurses, medicines, and food ... at any moment, night and day."

— Rufus Wyman, addressing the Trustees of the Massachusetts General Hospital, January 10, 1822

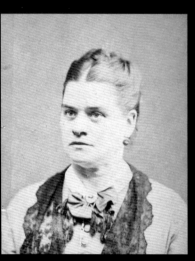 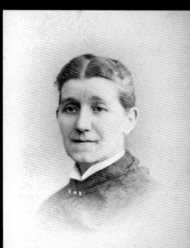 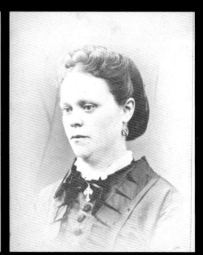

The images above are among the earliest photographs of MGH nurses. Pictured (l. to r.) are Mrs. Julia Sweeny, night nurse (who "came from Joy St." in the Beacon Hill section of Boston); Miss Crockett, charge of Surgical Ward 28; and Sarah Darrah, charge of Men's Ward in the Brick.

The Untrained Nurse

When the MGH first began admitting patients, the country was very young; the Revolutionary War had ended just 38 years prior. New York Hospital and Pennsylvania Hospital in Philadelphia were the only other hospitals in the United States, and there were no nursing schools. The hospital's nurses were virtually untrained, and early descriptions paint a dismal picture:

"Nurses were described as being of the poorest grade, women such as you would not have admitted to your own household, but some of them were kind and good. They had no teaching, just what they could pick up by experience or listening to the doctors, and the patients were cared for by rule of thumb. If the nurse was kind the nursing was fairly well done; if not, the patient was neglected.

"Cleanliness was not specially considered, and the wards were often dirty. ... The whole hospital had a peculiar hospital smell.

"The night nursing was very poor, only one woman to a large part of the hospital, and the patients got along as they could, and helped each other, but there was a great lack of proper care and discipline. ... There were occasional cases of drunken nurses and accidents arising therefrom. The wages of a hospital nurse were $2.00 a week.

"Among these ordinary nurses there shone out some who were born to the work and have never had their superiors as fine nurses and comforters of the sick."

— The Quarterly Record *of the MGH Nurses' Alumnae Association*

13

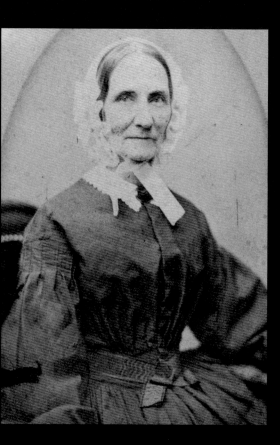

On November 10, 1860, Dr. J. Mason Warren requested that the hospital Trustees place the above portrait of Miss Rebecca Taylor in the Trustees Room. On the back, he wrote, "For 34 years a nurse at the Mass. General Hospital. Was 60 years of age when she left the hospital in Oct. 1860. Had the charge during the 34 years of 4,000 patients. Given to the Hospital by J. Mason Warren."

In an introductory lecture to the medical class of Harvard University on November 6, 1867, Oliver Wendell Holmes stated, "A clinical dialogue between Dr. Jackson and Miss Rebecca Taylor … was as good questioning and answering as one would like to hear outside of a courtroom."

Rebecca Taylor's contributions were widely recognized, as evidenced by the actions of the hospital's Trustees. On October 12, 1860, the Board voted "that in consideration of the advanced age of Miss Taylor, and her long and faithful services as nurse, which are held in grateful remembrance by the Trustees, she be relieved from all duties to the Hospital, and that her wages be continued till further order of the Board."

In a separate tribute to this early legendary nurse, Dr. James Jackson eloquently described the "high duties" of nursing — observations as apt today as they were in the 19th century. He also includes an informative exemplar, of sorts:

"I am tempted to take this occasion to put in print a statement of the merits of a nurse in the Massachusetts General Hospital, who began her career there a few years after it was opened, and after a service of thirty-four years, left that excellent institution a few months since.

"Miss Rebecca Taylor sought employment for her living. Having gained an appointment, she gave herself to her duties.

"She must have had system and industry, for I always found her work was done in proper season. Her fidelity, her tenderness, her patience, were proved by the uniform satisfaction shown by the sick under her care. Everything about her shows calmness and composure of mind. She uses few words, but they are apposite, very definite, and are uttered distinctly. …

us a very satisfactory account of the case from day to day, and with her intervention the management of the case was so successful, that the patient was dismissed well after a week or two.

"Meanwhile our Dutch woman learned to speak two words of imperfect English, which she repeated daily, pointing to our Miss Taylor. These

---

"A clinical dialogue between Dr. Jackson and Miss Rebecca Taylor … was as good a questioning and answering as one would like to hear outside of a courtroom."

"Many years ago there was placed in Miss Taylor's ward a very respectable Dutch woman, who had recently arrived in this country, and could not speak a word of English. … As none of us could speak in the Dutch tongue, we obtained help from two learned Germans; but after four or five days, we were able to relieve them from further attendance. Miss Taylor had established a language of signs with the patient, and watched her so closely, that she was able to give

words were 'too goot, too goot.'

"I have always known how difficult the duty of a nurse is; how much it requires to make a good one. … I avail myself gladly of an opportunity to leave behind me this testimony to her merits. … And, I will add, that, so far as my influence can go, I wish to point out how high are the duties of a nurse; and how justly they entitle one, who performs them skillfully and faithfully and kindly, to the love and respect of mankind."

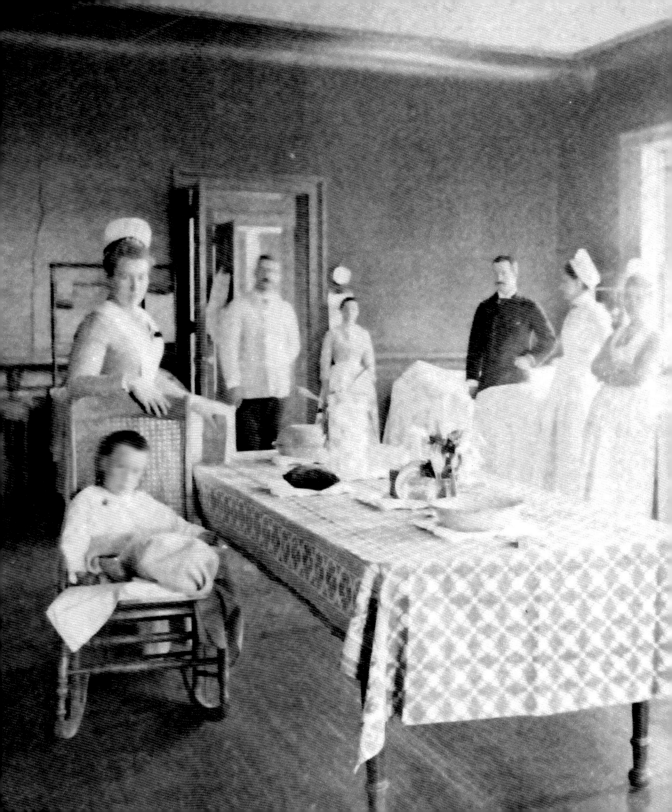

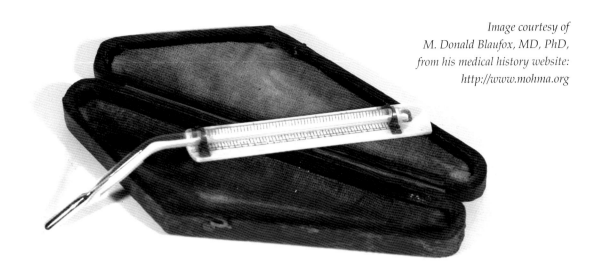

Image courtesy of M. Donald Blaufox, MD, PhD, from his medical history website: http://www.mohma.org

"The thermometers were large, clumsy things which bent at right angles and which had to be left in the axilla fifteen minutes before the temperature could be read and then it must be read before removing the thermometer. It was indeed discouraging when a patient, wishing to help the nurse, upon seeing her go towards the bed would take out the thermometer, hand it to the nurse, and say with a smile, 'There, nurse, I have taken it out to help you.' There was nothing left for the hurried and often tired nurse to do but to take the thermometer and replace it for another fifteen minutes. These were very precious articles, costing five dollars, and nurses when unfortunate enough to break one had half the price to pay. But even that, to nurses in training, if indulged in very much, became a very expensive pleasure and only a very reliable patient was allowed to hold the thermometer by herself."

— *Linda Richards,* American Journal of Nursing

Mary Elizabeth Norris was a nurse at the MGH from 1861 to 1868. At age 93, during an interview conducted by then assistant director of Nursing Ruth Sleeper, she recalled the working conditions and sparse training associated with her earlier career.

"We had no preparation for nursing in those days. I had never been inside a hospital. I was only 18 years old. We wore no uniform, just a simple dress.

"I came to Ward 23 feeling very much frightened. The first thing I had to do was set the table for the patients' dinner. We had two large tables on the Ward, and the patients who were up sat at one table. There was no kitchen on the Ward. The food was brought up by a man from the hospital kitchen downstairs. The nurse carried the dishes to the kitchen on a large wooden tray when she went for her own meals. With the help of a kind patient, I found the silver and dishes and set the table. Patients had to be carried up and down long flights of stairs … as I was leaving, an elevator was to be installed.

"The day nurses began work at five o'clock in the morning, had breakfast at seven o'clock, and finished their day's work at 10 o'clock at night. The pay was $9 a month for assistant head nurse and $13 a month for head nurse.

"The nurses slept in a little room between the wards. There was a double sofa in the clothes closet in the room. In the morning we would get up, put away the bedding and fold up the sofa. The room was then ready to be used as a thoroughfare between Wards 23 and 29.

"I was assistant head nurse on Ward 23 for about a year in 1861. Then Dr. Shaw, who was superintendent of the hospital, called me to his office and asked me how I should like to be head nurse. I told him I did not know enough, that I did not know how to be a head nurse; but he asked me to try it, and so I was head nurse on Ward 29 from '62 to '68. I was there during the [Civil] War.

"There were 21 patients on Ward 29.

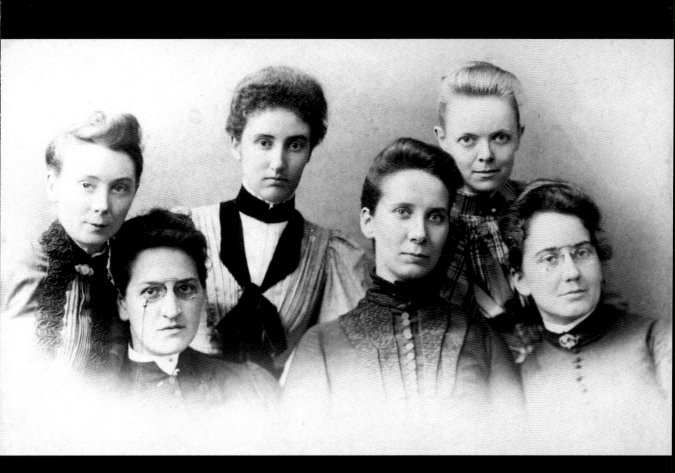

Early MGH nurses

I had one assistant and sometimes two. A ward tender gave the baths to the Men's Ward. The doctors did all the dressings. The nurses swept, dusted, made the beds, and gave baths. The head nurse gave medicines and was responsible for the diets. There were no classes; one nurse taught another what she knew. ... As a head nurse of Ward 29, every two weeks I had to send up a tray to the operating room. On it were bandages, compresses, hot oil, and a pin cushion with the needles in it. The ward tender got the instruments out of the case and spread them on the table. After the operation the nurse cleaned up the room and carried the bloodstained bandages and linen to the rinse house, where she rinsed all the blood out before sending it to the laundry."

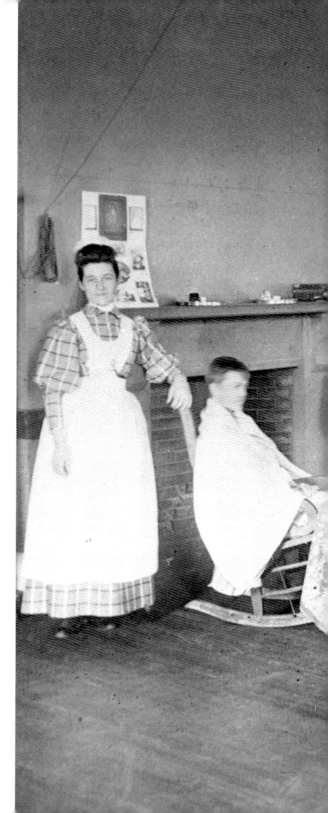

Ward 29 Surgical, Bulfinch Building, c. 1900
Head nurse Miss Bangs stands by the chimney.

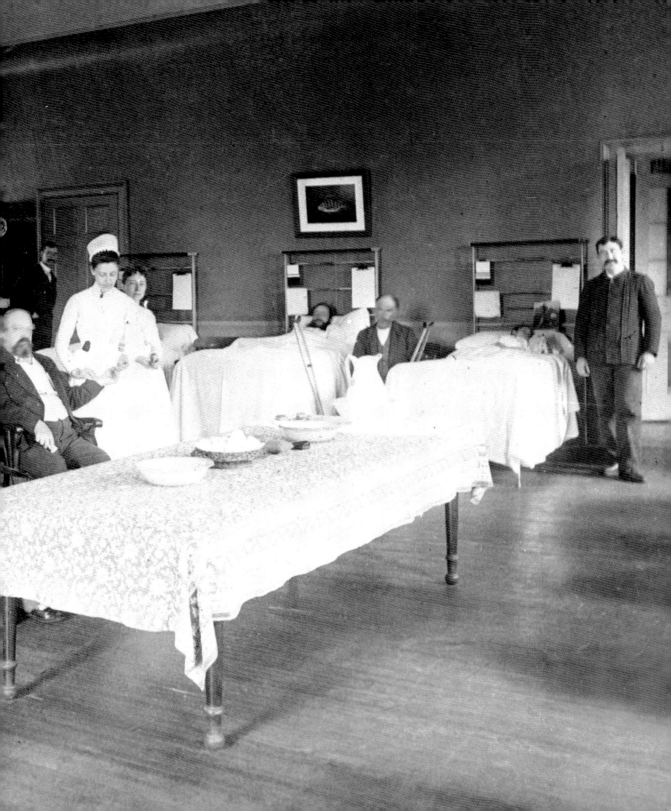

Emily Elizabeth Parsons

From 1861 to 1862, years before nursing education was available in the United States, Emily Elizabeth Parsons of Cambridge, Mass., spent 18 months at the MGH under the tutelage of two of its surgeons, Drs. Warren and Townshend. Although she never formally worked at the MGH, she was preparing herself for service in the Civil War. Some of her accomplishments are recorded on a plaque that hangs in the foyer of the Parsons Building at Mount Auburn Hospital, originally known as Cambridge Hospital:

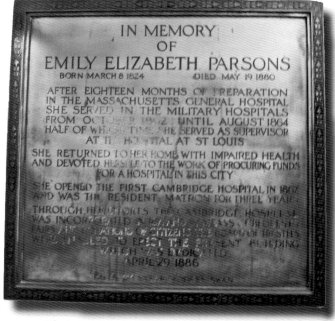

Photo courtesy of Mount Auburn Hospital

"In Memory of Emily Elizabeth Parsons, born March 8, 1824, died May 18, 1880. After eighteen months of preparation in the Massachusetts General Hospital, she served in military hospitals from October 1862 until August 1864. Half of this time she served as supervisor at the hospital at St. Louis. She returned to her home with impaired health and devoted herself to the work of procuring funds for a hospital in this city. She opened the first Cambridge Hospital in 1867 and was the resident matron for three years. Through her efforts the Cambridge Hospital was incorporated in 1871, and by means of bequests, fairs and donations of citizens, the Board of Trustees was enabled to erect the present building which was dedicated April 29, 1886."

Sarah J. Wry served as the head nurse for Dr. Folsom's private rooms, and was a nurse in the hospital for upwards of 18 years. When she died in the winter of 1874, the Trustees desired to express their respect for her character and services, and their sense of loss that the institution, and all connected with it, had sustained in her death.

"Her labors were remarkable not only for their length and their fidelity, but still more for their gentleness and their refinement. Such quietness, such delicacy, such dignity as hers, are seldom combined with such efficiency in nursing. The patient who would take food from no other hand, took it from hers, and when no one else could calm him, she would soothe him and induce him to sleep. She had the power to dispel much of the sadness which attaches to a sick bed, particularly in the wards of a hospital, and where she came some sort of cheerfulness always followed. Her moral influence over any a patient went further towards bringing about recovery than any other means she used. It sprang not from her manner or her words alone, but from her life. …

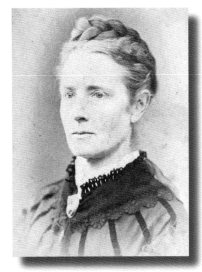

Sarah J. Wry

"In the death of such a nurse, the Trustees feel that the Hospital has met with a great bereavement. One of its oldest, one of its most faithful and helpful friends has been taken away, and the place she leaves must long be empty. The Trustees assume the expenses of her funeral as but part of the tribute due a career so long, so successful and so completely honorable. It is their privilege to bear witness to her as they have known her, and to remember her, in the way she would most wish to be remembered, as the Good Nurse."

Georgia Sturtevant began work as assistant head nurse of Ward 23 at the MGH in 1862. Two months later, she was appointed head nurse of Wards 29 and C at a salary of $13 per month. From 1869 to 1894, she served as matron, and earned a "very luxurious salary" of $17 per month. Sturtevant is regarded as the hospital's last untrained nurse, and her writings provide another glimpse of nursing in the 19th century.

"In 1862, the second year of our Civil War, I felt that I ought in some way to take part in that great struggle, and about decided to offer my services as an army nurse, but my friends persuaded me to abandon that idea, and remain at home. I accordingly gave up my army plans, and accepted a position as assistant nurse in the Massachusetts General Hospital, at a salary of $7.50 per month. ...

"I went into hospital work with no poetic ideas about nursing; I was fully prepared for hard, disagreeable duties, and for long, tedious days. ... I was not, however, prepared for the drudgery that was required of a hospital under-nurse in those days. I refer especially to the washing of filthy clothing and foul dressings that the assistant nurses had to do. ...

"I think the most uncharitable must give those women credit for some nobler inspiration, to keep alive their enthusiasm, than the $7.50 a month which they received for their services [which was low even for the 1860s].

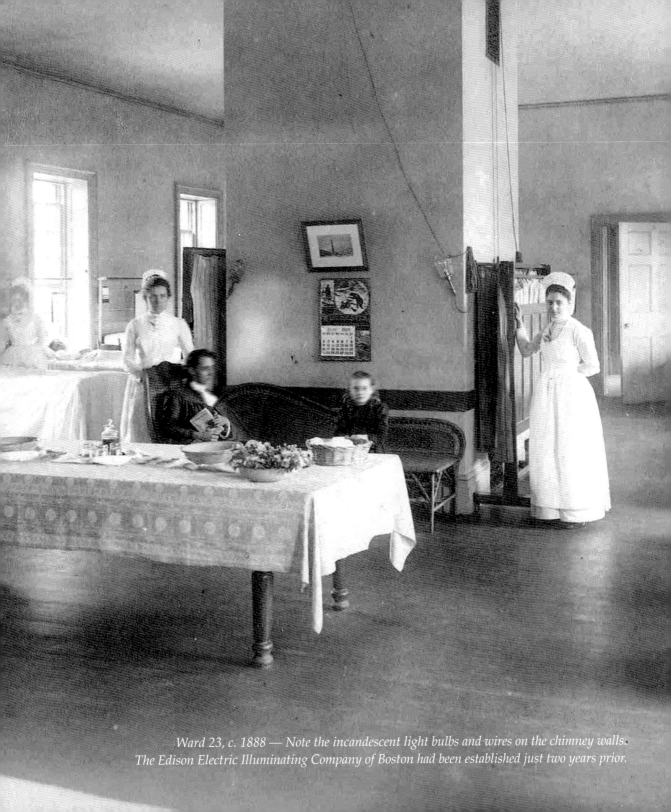

Ward 23, c. 1888 — Note the incandescent light bulbs and wires on the chimney walls.
The Edison Electric Illuminating Company of Boston had been established just two years prior.

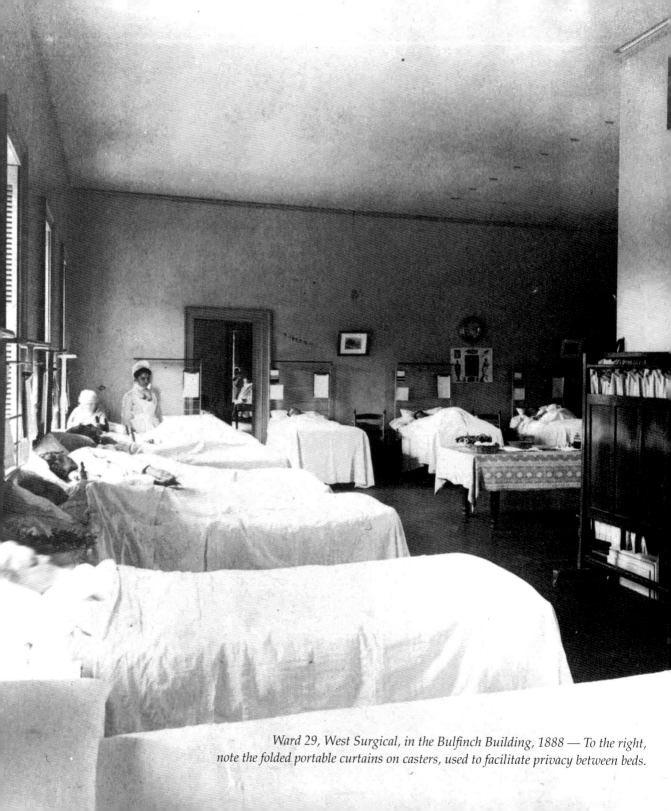

Ward 29, West Surgical, in the Bulfinch Building, 1888 — To the right, note the folded portable curtains on casters, used to facilitate privacy between beds.

Though the nurses received no special training, were given no systematic instruction, everything impressed me as being exceedingly systematic, and the smallest details important.

"After breakfast the assistant had the washing of the dishes to attend to, there being no ward maid, her sweeping and dusting to finish, and meanwhile assist the head nurse. ... Then came the rinsing of soiled clothing, the washing and ironing of bandages, etc. ... All the mending for the wards was done by the nurses, or the convalescent patients.

"Instead of conning [learning] her lessons or attending lectures, as the nurse of today [1895] has the privilege of doing, the nurse of that time, after attending to the wants of her patients, sat in her little room between the wards and patched the hospital linen, and at the same time on the alert for the calls that were sure to come from time to time from the ward outside. ...

"These may seem unnecessary and unimportant details, but I give them to show some of the difficulties that women encountered who desired to get an education in nursing thirty years ago. ... Some of these women would gladly have devoted their whole time to the better care of the patients and for their own instruction as well, instead of wasting it in those menial offices which should have been delegated to laundry women, but which, for some unexplained reason, were strangely enough included in the duties of a nurse.

"One of these results [of the war] was to bring our hospitals more prominently before the public, and call urgently for the much needed improvement, not only in their construction and organization, but in providing facilities for educating women in the art of nursing the sick. An art, which up to that time, they had apparently been supposed to know by intuition, and were blamed for their ignorance if they failed in some point, and were reprimanded rather unpleasantly if they knew *too much*."

A 19th Century Exemplar

Written by Miss Georgia Sturtevant,
a nurse at Massachusetts General Hospital from 1862 to 1894
The Trained Nurse, *April 1896*

"Human nature is a complex problem at best, and sick human nature is sometimes incomprehensible. A nurse has two distinct conditions to consider—the individual and the case. She has not only to watch the physical symptoms, but the moods, and frequently the personal eccentricities of the patient as well, and sometimes the latter is much the hardest task of all. She is always in a state of expectancy; always on the alert for some new development.

"Sometimes tokens of gratitude, in the form of kind words, come back to her from appreciative patients or their friends, and again, where she has done the most and endured the most, she receives only censure.

"Willie C, a poor, haggard, emaciated boy, worn out and fractious by long years of sickness and intense suffering, was brought to the hospital. We looked upon him as a boy, though against his name we read 'Age 22.' The case was that of a 'bad knee' and it proved to be very bad indeed, and after some weeks of treatment, it finally came to amputation. It was a long, tedious case, and the nurses were quite worn out with Willie's almost ceaseless, fretful demands upon them during the many weeks that lengthened into months that he was under our care. Even the patience of his mother, who had remained with him for a time, was finally exhausted and she left him in our hands.

"But there came a day [about six months later] when Willie was discharged. We brought out his clothes and we brushed his hair, and put on his one shoe. We wrapped him in warm blankets, and the strong ward tender took him in his arms to the carriage, and as the carriage drove out of the hospital grounds we drew a breath of relief. Yes, we were glad that Willie was gone, and yet we were sorry that we were glad.

"[After he had gone] we missed his peevish calls, and his pale face haunted us. We would ask ourselves, 'I wonder if we were patient enough with Willie?' and then the consoling thought would come, 'But even his mother got out of patience with him.' And we would fall asleep, to be wakened by the night watcher's call, 'Quarter of five!'

"No tidings came back to us of Willie. But a reckoning day came when we least expected it. 'A gentleman in the reception-room to see you,' was announced one morning by the porter [five years later], and an uncomfortable presentiment of coming disaster took possession of me. I arranged my hair with trembling fingers—no caps in those days, unfortunately, to give dignity to one's bearing and confidence as a badge of office will—for even a nurse, an untrained nurse, cannot control her emotions under all circumstances. I went down the long flight of stone stairs, and as I opened the door of the reception room a gentleman advanced to meet me. His stern face added greatly to my discomfiture, and my self-control nearly deserted me. The gentleman asked, 'Are you Miss ------, and did you have the care of a patient by the name of Willie C? Was he very troublesome?'

"I answered in the affirmative as calmly as I was able. The picture of indignant parents, sympathizing friends, and the 'family physician,' whom I had every reason to believe was standing before me, passed rapidly before my mind. But though my hands had grown absolutely clammy by this time, I determined to defend myself and regain my self-control by talking very rapidly, and I answered, 'Yes, he certainly was very troublesome indeed. We knew that he had suffered a long time, and we really pitied the boy very much, and we tried to be very patient with him, but his fretfulness did at times seem almost unbearable. Even his mother—'

"But what a remarkable change had come over the stranger. His stern features had softened and a smile transformed his face, as he answered, 'Yes, even my mother couldn't stand my nonsense. For I am Willie C, and I have come back to apologize for my bad behavior.' And he held out his hand, and I noticed for the first time the artificial leg that he had learned to manage with perfect ease. Here indeed was a case of gratitude we were wholly unprepared for."

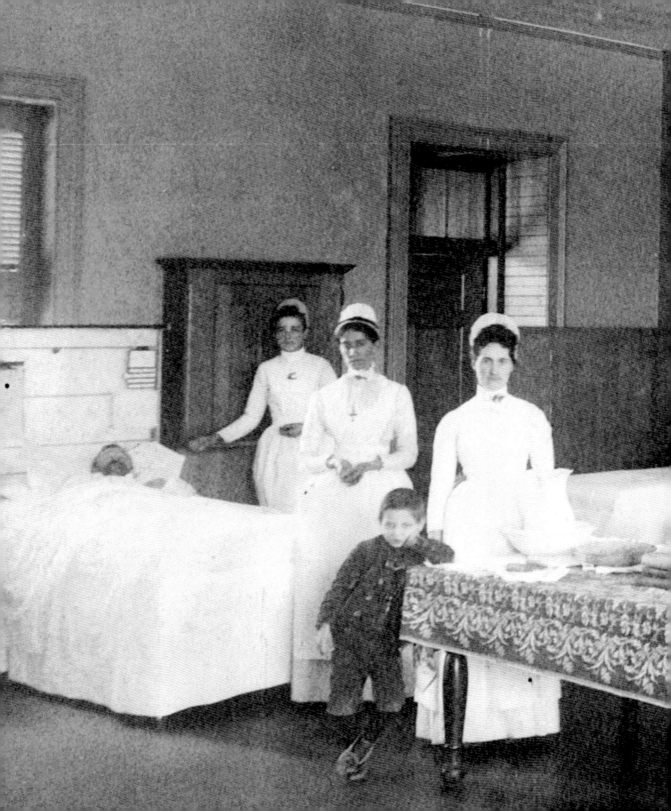

The Trained Nurse

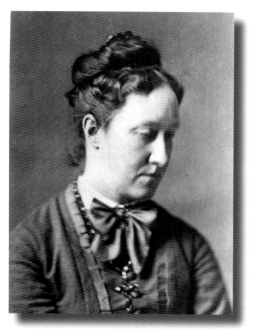

Miss Sarah Cabot

In 1872, the Industrial Committee of the Woman's Education Association in Boston brought together a group of visionaries who played a critical role in establishing nursing education in the United States. The Association was seeking new occupations for self-supporting women. Miss Sarah Cabot, whose brother was a physician at MGH, suggested establishing a training school for nurses.

At the time no such school existed in the country, but Miss Cabot, a director at the New England Hospital for Women and Children, knew of a nurse training program being started there. She consulted with Mrs. Samuel Parkman, who was enthusiastic, as she had recently met Florence Nightingale on a visit to England and learned of her system of training.

Miss Cabot and Mrs. Parkman recruited a group of ladies and gentlemen, who met at the Parkman home throughout the winter to explore the idea. In April 1873, the Association recommended creating a formal committee to develop a plan, thereby ending its ties to the effort; the committee was now functioning independently. In May, the members wrote to the MGH Trustees: "The undersigned propose to establish in Boston a Training School for Nurses, which shall furnish for hospitals and private families a better

School of Nursing in New York City was established, becoming the country's first school of nursing using the Nightingale model, followed a few short months later by the Connecticut

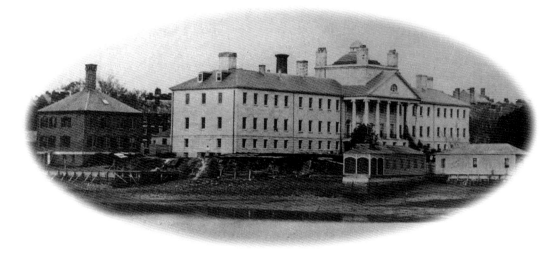

To the left of the Bulfinch Building is "the Brick" or "Foul Ward," where the hospital's first student nurses were assigned.

class of nurses than can now be obtained. They believe that a carefully guided apprenticeship and an intelligent oversight will do much to raise the standard of ability and fidelity, and that personal sympathy and a good organization may adjust in leading women to look upon nursing as a desirable profession."

That same month, the Bellevue Hospital

Training School for Nurses in New Haven and the Boston Training School for Nurses at MGH. With the exception of Miss Cabot's brother, most of the physicians at the MGH, including Benjamin S. Shaw, the resident physician, were not in favor of a school for nurses, nor were many of the Trustees.

According to Miss Cabot's account, "After some talk they consented, reluctantly, to let us try our experiment in what was called the 'Foul Ward,' a very undesirable part of the hospital occupied by cancer cases and delirium tremens; having found it hard to manage themselves, they were willing to let us try."

With just four applicants, the Boston Training School for Nurses started at Massachusetts General Hospital on November 1, 1873. The school was to be run on a probationary period, with the Trustees able to sever the relationship at any time.

"Having prepared a list of subjects which we wished the doctors to lecture upon before the nurses of the training school, Mrs. Howland Shaw and I, carrying this list with us, visited all the doctors that we could reach, hoping to persuade them to oblige us by lecturing. We found that they manifested very little interest, though some were courteous enough to promise to do so because they were asked. However, on reaching Dr. Oliver Wendell Holmes, he voiced without hesitation, as I think, the feeling that most of the other doctors had. He didn't wish to do anything towards making these nurses feel too much their importance, or as he considered, they would be dangerous from a mistaken idea that they knew more than they really did."

The school's first year proved a struggle. Because the MGH physicians refused to lecture, the school's directors relied upon the staff of Boston City Hospital and other outside physicians for instruction. The first superintendent, Mrs. Billings, resigned after just three months. Her successor, Mrs. von Olnhausen, was described as "temperamentally … not well fitted" for the position. The pupils quickly caught up in knowledge with one of the head nurses, who eventually entered the school herself. For a time, the school's future was considered doubtful. Fortunately, the original committee members were highly regarded within the larger community, as well as by the hospital's physicians and Trustees. This alone may have prompted the hospital to agree to continue the school for another year. But they did so only under certain conditions, including the hiring a superintendent who was a trained nurse, of which there were only a handful in the country.

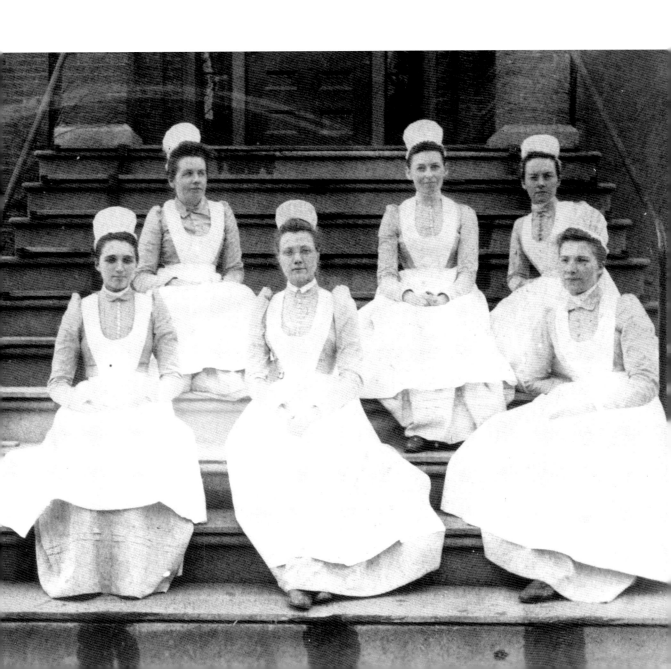

The hospital Trustees wanted a trained nurse in charge of the school, and the school's directors were fortunate to recruit Linda Richards, regarded as America's first trained nurse. She began her tenure as superintendent on November 1, 1874.

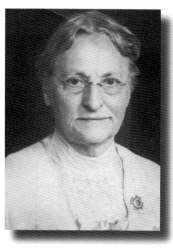

"It may prove of interest to describe just how the work was arranged there on my arrival. The hospital, although it was wealthy, was very economical in many ways. For instance, all poultice cloths which had no discharge upon them, and all the bandages which were considered clean, were washed and ironed by hand and used again. They might be washed several times. Now it fell to the lot of the nurses to do this washing, and I assure you it was all of that hard work.

"There was, moreover, the strangest division of labor. For instance, a nurse would begin a day by washing poultice cloths and bandages, and it would often be two o'clock before her work was finished. She then went off duty for the afternoon. The second day the same nurse helped in the dining room service and in washing dishes. After this was done, she was ready to do little incidental things as need arose. The third day she went into the wards, washed the patients' faces, made beds, swept floors, and did this, that, and the other duty until night. The fourth she would act as head nurse. The fifth day she would begin as general utility nurse, but at nine go off duty to sleep, so as to be ready to go on duty that night. The sixth day she had to herself. Then the same rotation of service began again.

"The doctors complained that nobody knew anything, and surely it was no wonder. We had many trials before order was brought out of confusion and a regular system finally settled upon.

"We at once began class instruction as

a regular part of the nurses' education, and very soon we changed the routine of work. At the end of this year I had nurses sufficiently well-trained to be intrusted [sic] with responsibilities, and the work of the superintendent was made easier. The school had increased in size, and served all the wards of the hospital, except that for private patients, a small ward of separate rooms.

transforming the institution into a premier nurse training program and creating a model for other such programs to follow. She brought much-needed order and purpose to training the nursing students — who at the time also served as the hospital's nursing staff — and the overall organization and quality of work improved. At the end of the first three months, the Trustees voted to

"The doctors complained that nobody knew anything, and surely it was no wonder. We had many trials before order was brought out of confusion and a regular system finally settled upon."

"From this time on, the hospital staff lectured to the nurses, and Dr. H. J. Bigelow began the practice of taking the nurses with him on his visits to the wards. Members of his staff frequently spoke of 'our school' with interest and pride. The change was marvelous."

Miss Richards is credited for

give Miss Richards and the students an additional ward.

With Linda Richards' leadership, the evolution of nursing as a profession began to emerge. She expanded the role of the nurses from the "Foul Ward" to being in charge of every ward in the hospital. She obtained a thermometer for the school and a textbook from the Connecticut Training School for Nurses in New Haven. She established regular class instruction for her pupils, who had previously only received infrequent lectures. She implemented cooking (nutrition) classes and transferred non-nursing duties to maids, allowing her students to spend more time with their patients. Richards also initiated the practice of keeping patient records at the bedside to be readily available to physicians and students. This was the first written reporting system for nurses, a practice that was later adopted by the Nightingale System.

Richards left the Boston Training School for Nurses in 1877 and spent several months in London and Edinburgh studying under Florence Nightingale before returning to the United States. She later spent five years as a medical missionary in Kyoto, Japan, where she established that country's first school of nursing.

Upon returning to the United States, she continued in many leadership roles, including serving as the first president of the American Society of Superintendents of Training Schools for nurses — the first professional organization for nurses — but for limited periods due to poor health.

In no small way, Linda Richards represents the birth of professional nursing, and today her certificate of graduation is housed at the Smithsonian Institution in Washington, D.C.

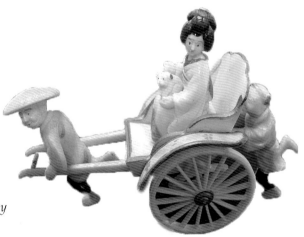

A figurine that once belonged to Linda Richards is today housed in the MGH Archives and Special Collections.

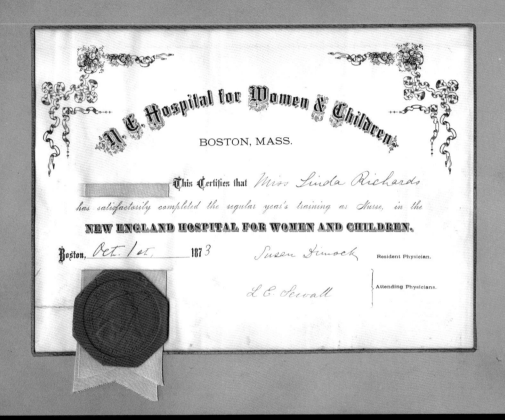

N. E. Hospital for Women & Children

BOSTON, MASS.

This Certifies that *Miss Linda Richards* has satisfactorily completed the regular year's training as Nurse, in the

NEW ENGLAND HOSPITAL FOR WOMEN AND CHILDREN,

Boston, *Oct. 1st*, 1873

Susan Dimock — Resident Physician.

L. C. Sewall — Attending Physicians.

In 1873, Linda Richards became the first student to enroll in and the first to graduate from a nurse training program offered at the New England Hospital for Women and Children. In doing so, she became America's first trained nurse. From 1874 to 1876, Richards served as the superintendent of the Boston Training School for Nurses, which was later renamed the Massachusetts General Hospital Training School for Nurses. She is credited with transforming the institution into one of the premier nurse training programs in the country. Photograph of Linda Richards' certificate of graduation, above, courtesy of the Division of Medicine & Science, National Museum of American History, Behring Center, Smithsonian Institution.

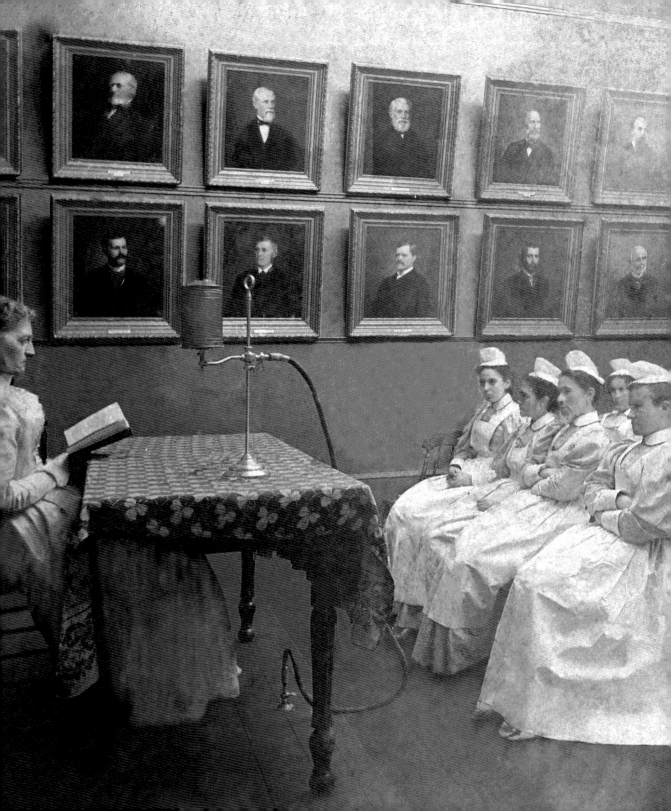

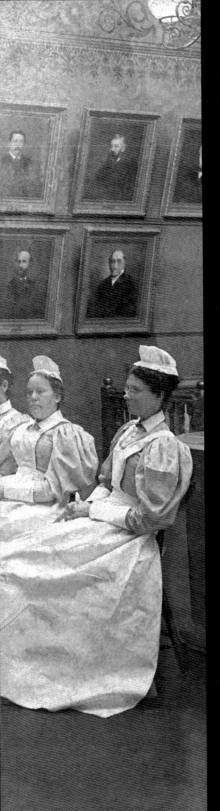

"*I have seldom seen anyone who struck me as so admirable. I think we have as much to learn from her as she has from us.*"

— *Florence Nightingale,*
introducing Linda Richards to the
matron of the Edinburgh Royal Infirmary

Pictured: Linda Richards instructs a classroom of nursing students.
From 1874 to 1877, Miss Richards served as superintendent of the
Boston Training School for Nurses, which was later renamed the
Massachusetts General Hospital Training School for Nurses.

The first documented use of nurses' caps is lost to history. Scholars debate whether they originated with the nursing sisters of religious orders, for whom caps were part of their attire, or in emulation of the cap worn by Florence Nightingale. During the Victorian era, it was customary to wear a cap while inside one's home; in a hospital setting, the cap denoted cleanliness and modesty.

Each hospital nursing school designed its own distinctive-looking cap, making their graduates easy to identify. The MGH introduced its first nursing cap in November 1878. A black velvet band on the cap denoted head nurse status. The earliest MGH caps were similar to those worn at New England Hospital for Women and Children, a reflection of MGH Training School Superintendent Anna Wollhampton's 1874 graduation from that school.

At first large and designed to cover the wearer's hair, these caps were made smaller and elongated in 1890, and underwent further changes in 1910 and 1922, gradually decreasing in size. Caps were never "formally" discontinued at MGH; they were worn for graduation ceremonies until the MGH School of Nursing closed in 1981, and some MGH graduates wore caps on the patient care units well into the 1980s.

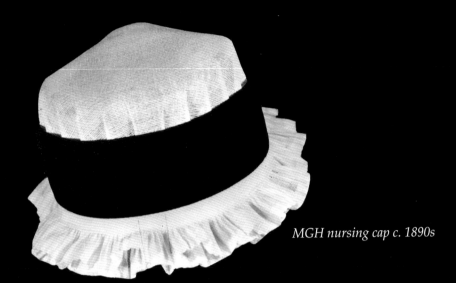

MGH nursing cap c. 1890s

The Massachusetts General Hospital School of Nursing pin

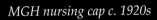 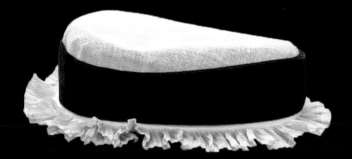

MGH nursing cap c. 1920s

As the patient load increased at the hospital, separate ward buildings were constructed. Connected by covered corridors, they were isolated from one another in an attempt to avoid infection transmittal. Known collectively as the Pavilion Wards, they were individually lettered and also named in recognition of prominent MGH physicians.

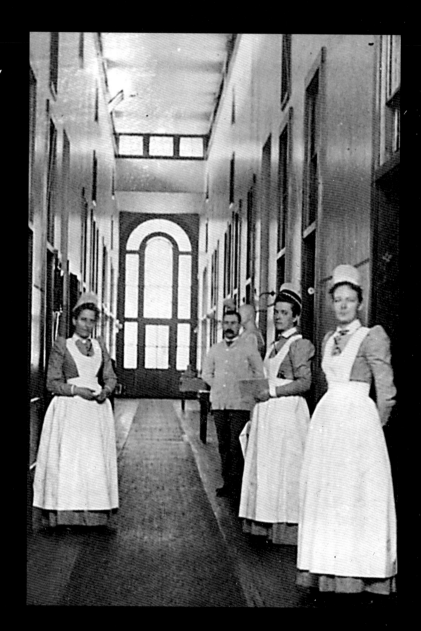

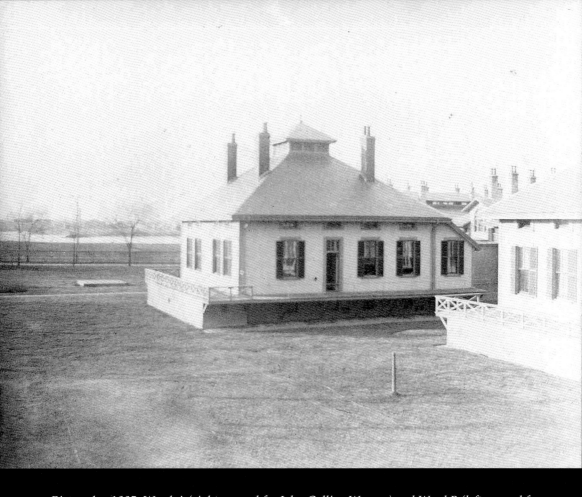

Pictured c. 1885, Ward A (right, named for John Collins Warren) and Ward B (left, named for James Jackson) were erected in 1873 as wooden pavilions designed on the model of Army field hospitals. They had several intended purposes, but they were primarily used as isolation wards for contagious cases. In the background is the Charles River.

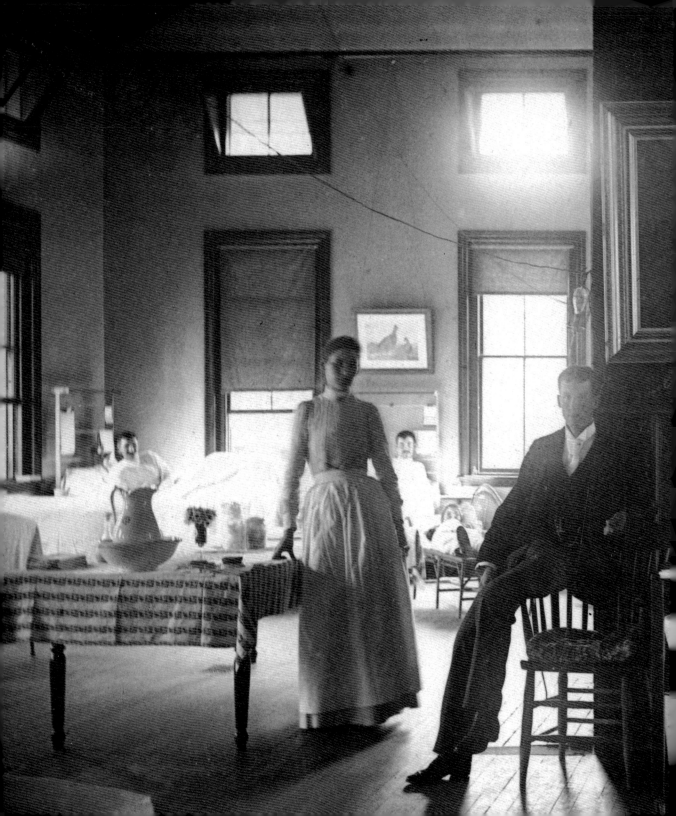

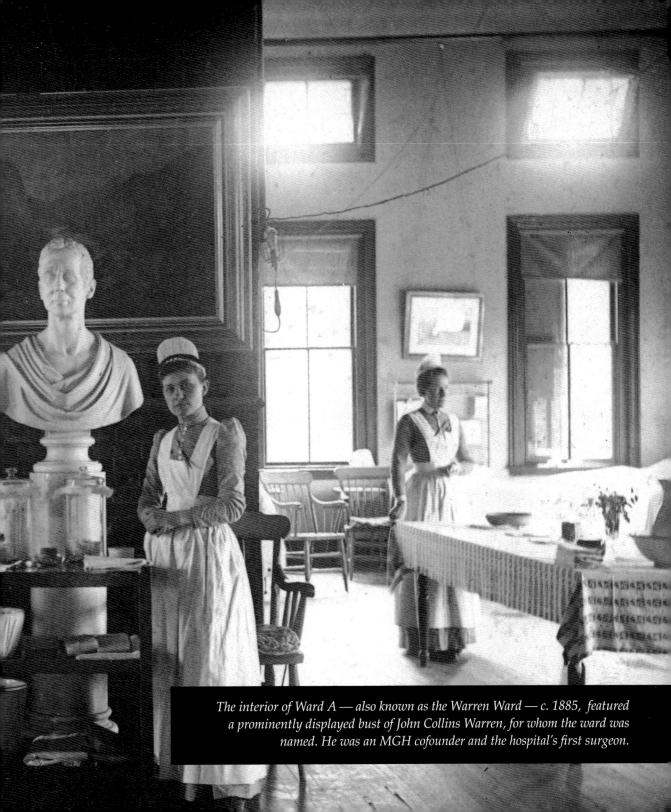

The interior of Ward A — also known as the Warren Ward — c. 1885, featured a prominently displayed bust of John Collins Warren, for whom the ward was named. He was an MGH cofounder and the hospital's first surgeon.

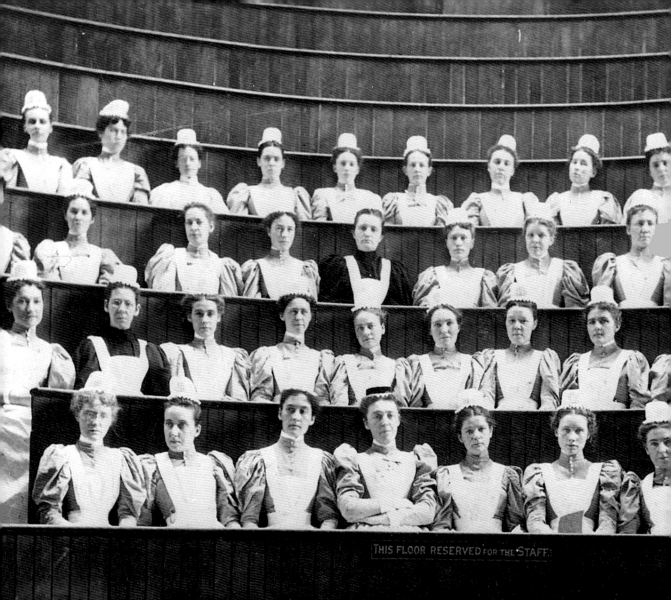

THIS FLOOR RESERVED FOR THE STAFF.

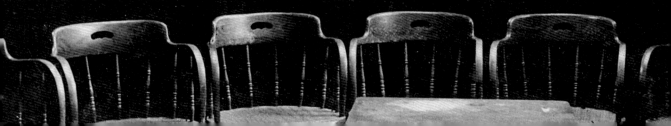

An undated photograph (c. late 1800s) shows a group of nursing students assembled in the Lower Outpatient Amphitheater. The night nurses can be identified by the dark-colored blouses they were required to wear. The instructor or head nurse (front row) is identified by a black band on her cap.

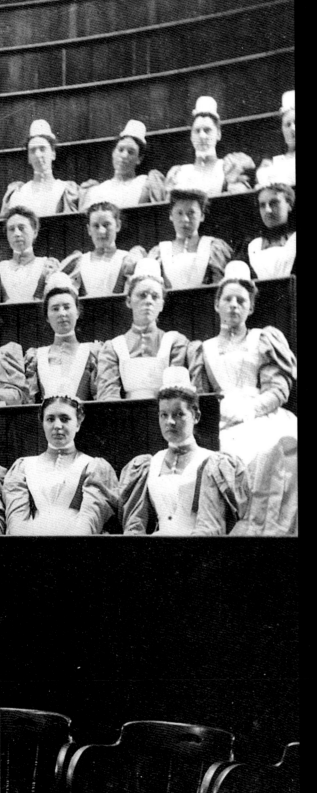

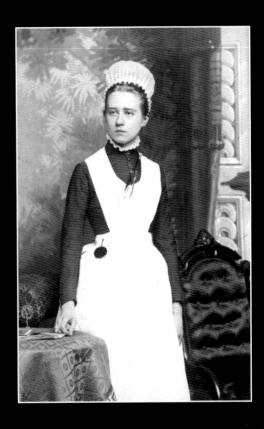

*Anna Palmberg, night nurse and 1888
graduate of the Boston Training School for
Nurses at Massachusetts General Hospital*

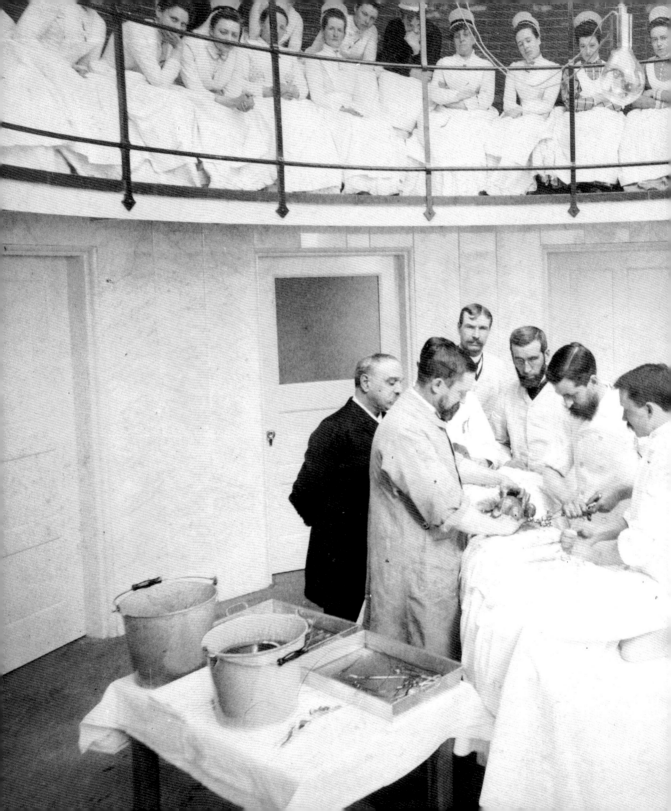

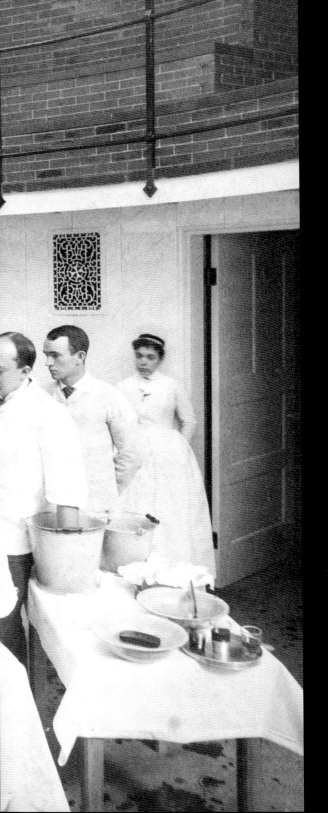

The Bradlee Ward Operating Theater for aseptic surgery, Ward E, 1889 — Dr. J. Collins Warren is operating, and Dr. Porter in his Prince Albert coat is looking over his shoulder. Mains, the operating room orderly, is standing at the head of the table, sporting a close-cropped beard. Conner, another orderly, stands in front of the nurse in attendance, Mary E. Melville, class of 1888. Note the simple equipment to do a laparotomy.

Nurses in gallery (l. to r.): fourth nurse, Mary Keith (class of 1888); behind post, Imogene Slade (1885); behind Miss Slade, Maria B. Brown (1883); seventh nurse, Isaline A. Davis (1885); next to third post, Mrs. Clark, head nurse of Ward B; next to fourth post, Carrie D. Bangs (1888)

Curriculum 1885: Lectures by Doctors

Typhoid Fever	*Dr. Abbott*
Rheumatic Fever	*Dr. Abbott*
Drugs and Preparation of Drugs	*Dr. Harrington*
Food: Kind, Preparation and Method of Giving	*Dr. Cabot*
Convulsions and Hemorrhages	*Dr. Cabot*
Administration of Medicine	*Dr. Cabot*
Treatment of Croup and Diphtheria	*Dr. Cabot*
Care of Patients with Nervous Diseases	*Dr. Putnam*
Massage	*Dr. Putnam*
Monthly Nursing (Care of Women in Confinement) (six lectures)	*Dr. Richardson*
Anaesthesia (two lectures)	*Dr. Richardson*
The Sick Room	*Dr. Shattuck*
Infectious Disease and the Care of the Patient	*Dr. Shattuck*
Care of Children (two lectures)	*Dr. Shattuck*
Private Nursing	*Dr. Shattuck*
Food and Feeding	*Dr. West*
Fractures	*Dr. West*
Bandages and Splints	*Dr. West*
Surgical Dressings, Plasters, Bed Sores	*Dr. West*
Urine	*Dr. West*
Skin	*Dr. White*
Afflictions of the Skin (two lectures)	*Dr. White*
The Eye	*Dr. Standish*
Care of the Dead and the Autopsy (three lectures)	*Dr. Cutler*
Secretions and Excretions	*Dr. Cutler*

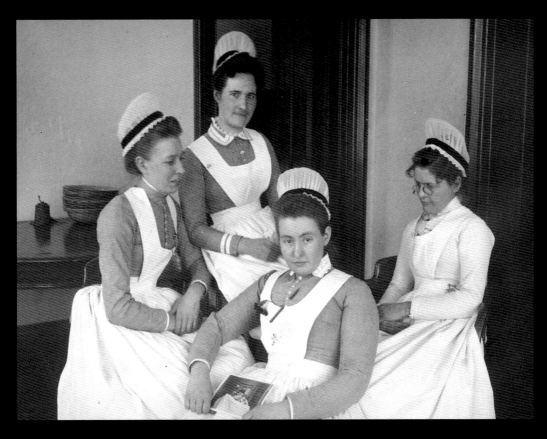

Pictured (l. to r.) c. 1890 are MGH head nurses Miss Smith; Miss Margaret Beckingham (1885); Miss Maria Brown (1883) superintendent of Nurses, 1889-1899; and Miss Parker.

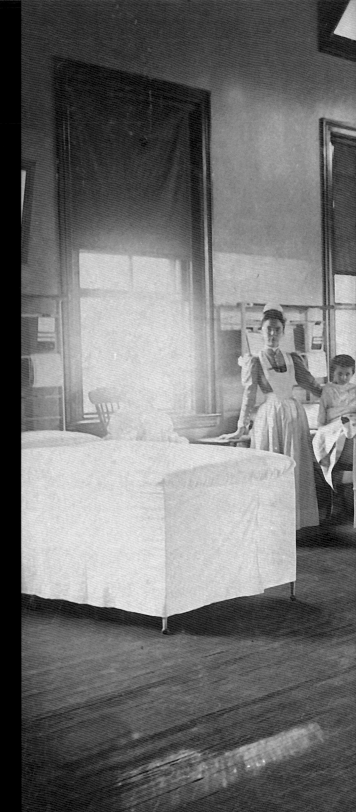

The sick room must be
ventilated. ... Poisonous
matter is constantly being
thrown off by the skin and
lungs, and if this poison
remains in the room it is
reabsorbed by the system and
does almost as much harm as
if it is poison administered by
mouth with a teaspoon."

— *Elisabeth Robinson Scovil,*
class of 1880,
The Care of Children, *1894*

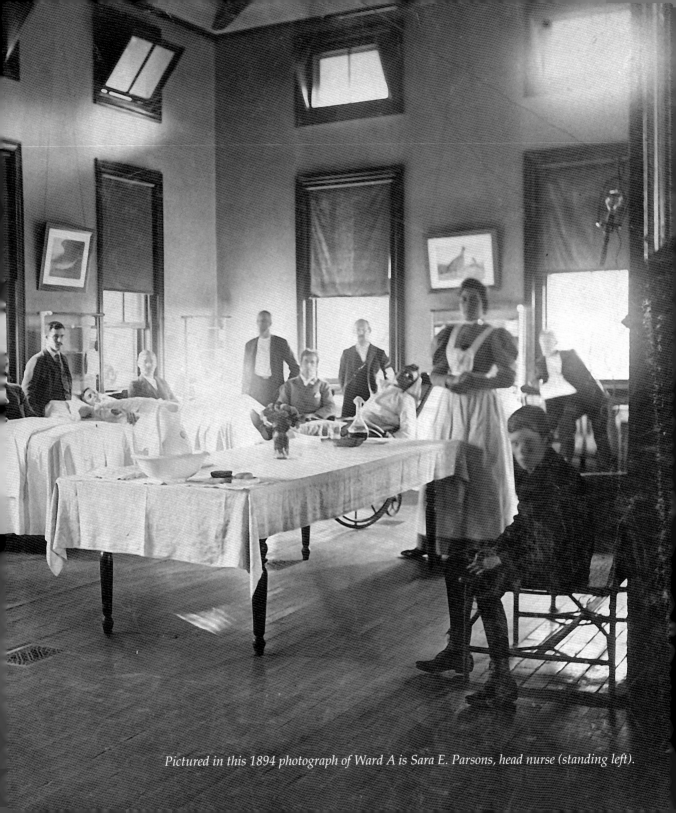

Pictured in this 1894 photograph of Ward A is Sara E. Parsons, head nurse (standing left).

HISTORY

OF THE

ALUMNÆ ASSOCIATION

OF THE

Boston and Massachusetts General Hospital

Hospital

TRAINING SCHOOL FOR NURSES,

On February 14, 1895, Miss Mary E.P. Davis and Miss Sophia F. Palmer, both class of 1878, started the Alumnae Association of the Boston Training School for Nurses, located at the Massachusetts General Hospital. There were 81 charter members of the Association. In the fall of 1896, delegates from 10 alumnae associations, including that of the MGH School, met to organize a national association, and the Nurses' Associated Alumnae of the United States and Canada began its work the next year. The first MGH delegate to the National Association was Miss Margaret W. Stevenson, class of 1890, and from that time until the closing of the school in 1981, a delegate was sent to the annual convention each year. In 1911, the organization officially took over ownership of the *American Journal of Nursing* and became the American Nurses Association.

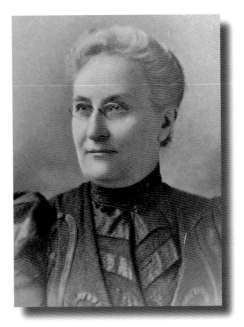

Mary E.P. Davis

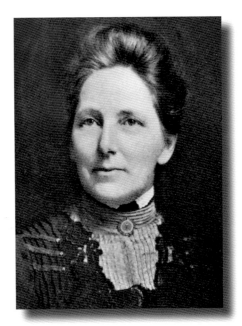

Sophia French Palmer

Nursing education slowly gained legitimacy and became an essential component of the developing American hospital. Nursing care offered by students provided the hospital with an inexpensive and essential labor force to fuel hospital growth in the 20th century.

In January of 1896, the hospital assumed ownership of the Boston Training School, merging it with the Nursing Service. The school was renamed the Massachusetts General Hospital Training School for Nurses and placed under the management of the MGH Trustees. The head of the Training School and the Nursing Service were one and the same.

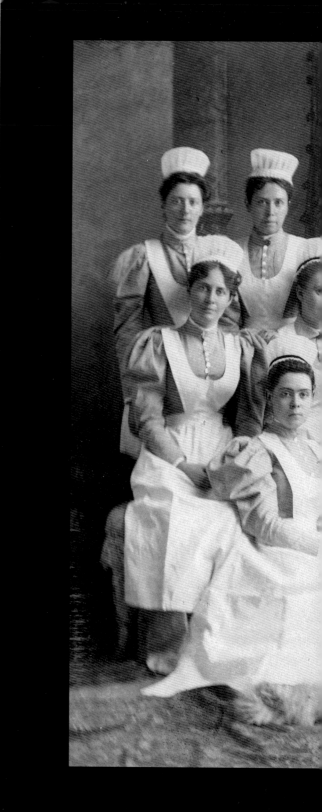

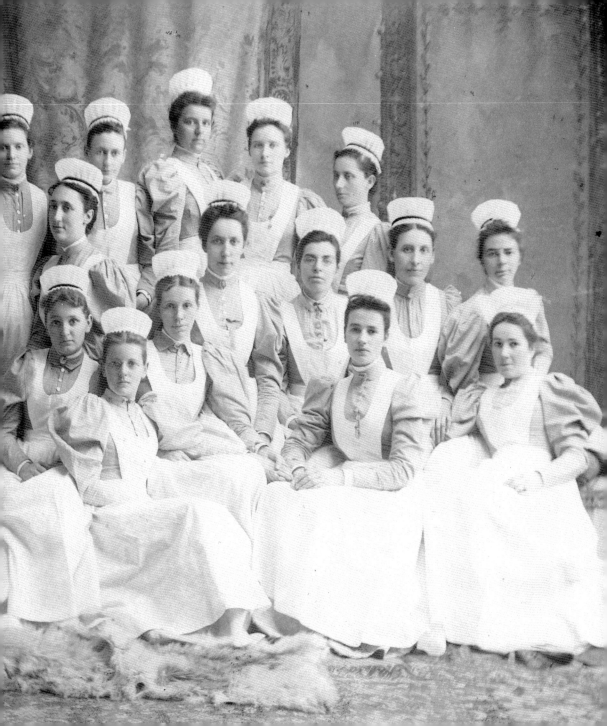

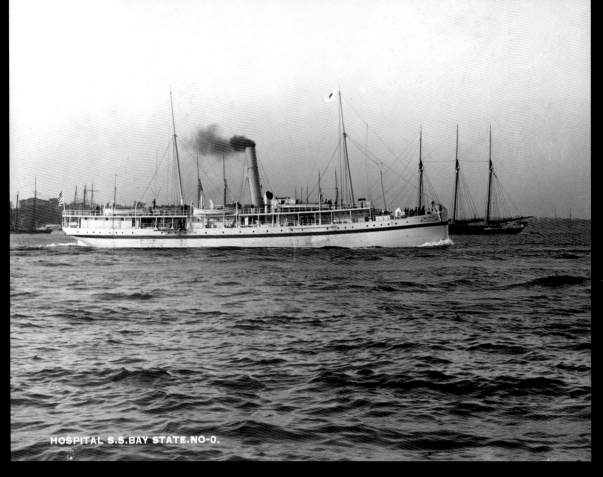

HOSPITAL S.S.BAY STATE.NO-0.

Photo shows the S.S. Bay State leaving Boston Harbor for Cuba, August 6, 1898. Image courtesy of the Massachusetts Historical Society.

In 1898, as the Spanish-American War continued, the people of Massachusetts rallied to equip a hospital ship to care for its soldiers, the only state to initiate such an effort. The *Bay State* was purchased with funds raised by the citizens of Massachusetts and outfitted by the Massachusetts Volunteer Aid Association. On June 23, 1898, President William McKinley officially signed the commission of the ship to aid the medical authorities of the Army and Navy in caring for the sick and wounded soldiers and sailors. This was the first hospital ship in the world to be fitted out by an aid association and authorized by a sovereign power under the articles of the Geneva Conference.

On August 6, the *Bay State* left Boston Harbor for Cuba loaded with provisions, two surgeons and six nurses, among them MGH Training School graduates Sara Parsons (1893), Muriel Galt (1898) and Mary B. Hall (1883). They carried everything needed to care for the soldiers from Massachusetts and bring them safely home. Between August and October, the ship made three round trips, first to Santiago, Cuba, then twice to Puerto Rico, bringing 336 sick and wounded soldiers back to Boston. Five patients died en route.

When the ship arrived in Boston, ambulances were waiting at the dock to transport the patients. Due to overcrowding, those brought home in the warmer months were cared for in tents on the hospital grounds. In addition to wounds suffered in battle, the patients also suffered from typhoid, dysentery, malaria, diarrhea, yellow fever and various other diseases.

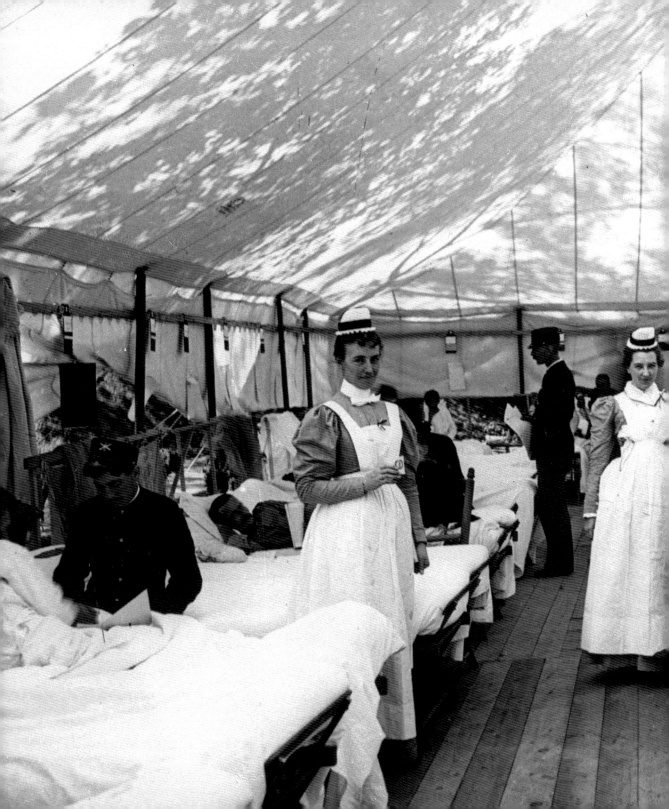

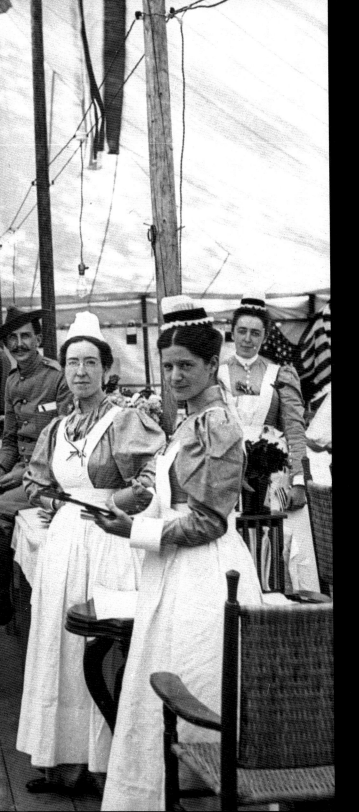

In 1898, during the Spanish-American War, the MGH accepted patients who were suffering from typhoid fever and malaria contracted in the subtropical climate of Cuba and Puerto Rico. A tent ward was erected on the Bulfinch Lawn, and nurses were assigned to care for these patients. Most recovered and were able to go home.

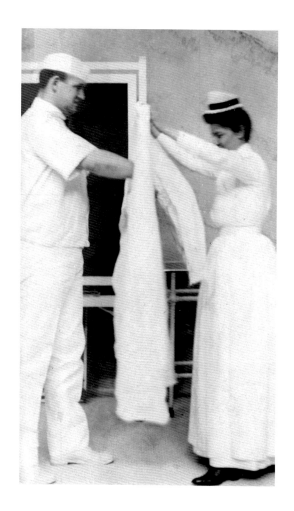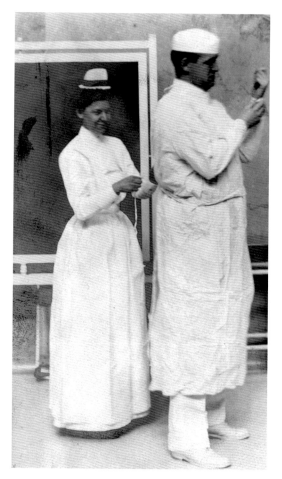

MGH instituted antiseptic surgical practices c. 1877. Seen here are two stages of "scrubs" in preparation for performing surgery, c. 1900. Although the English surgeon Joseph Lister's research suggested the need for asepsis as well as antisepsis in the operating room as early as the 1860s, many hospitals, including MGH, were slow to adjust. The MGH's first operating facility specifically designed for aseptic surgery, located in Bradlee Ward E, opened in 1888, making abdominal surgery safe from infection.

"The nurse who assisted the surgeon was referred to as the scrubbed (or scrub) nurse, suture nurse, instrument nurse, sterile glove nurse, or sponge nurse, among other names. Surgeons initially insisted that the scrub nurse be the most senior nurse, but eventually there was agreement by nurses that the unsterile or circulating nurse should be the most senior nurse."

— Comprehensive Perioperative Nursing,
Gruendemann and Fernsebner

The length of training in 1899 was still only two years, though by this time a two months' period of probation had been added at the beginning of the course. Once accepted into the School, students received six dollars each month for personal expenses.

Working hours for a month of night duty in 1899 were from 8 p.m. to 7 a.m. Day nurses worked from 6:45 a.m. to 8 p.m., with 20 to 30 minutes off for meals and one hour daily off duty. They also had a half-day off weekly in addition to four hours off on Sunday.

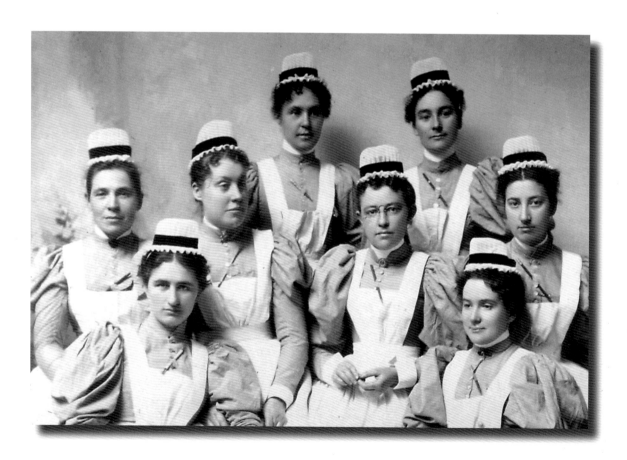

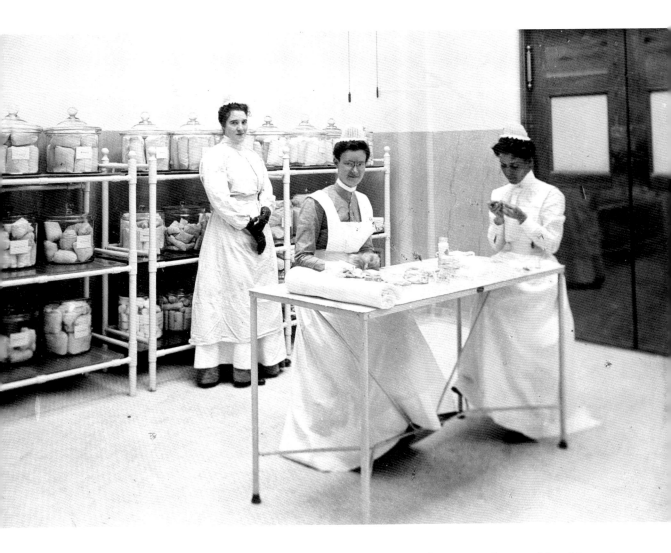

MGH nurses preparing bandages, c. 1900. In making bandages, it was usual to procure the material and to mark off the various widths required, varying from an inch for the fingers and toes to about four inches for the trunk. The length was usually about six yards. The strips were torn and wound either with the fingers or by a machine. In winding with the fingers, the bandage was wound evenly and tightly. All threads were removed from the edges, and the tail was secured either with a pin or a few threads wound round the roller. Where many were required, a bandage roller became useful. One end of the bandage was fixed round the central rod, not too tightly, or the roller could not easily be removed. The handle was then turned, and the bandage was wound evenly and firmly.

In 1903, the annual report of the hospital's visiting staff refers to a discussion about the policy of using house officers to administer anesthesia. The recommendation was for "the establishment of paid nurse anaesthetists, one for each surgical service." Although MGH was not the first to do so, it was early in introducing nurses to the field of anesthesia.

Helen Altimus and Grace Perkins, both class of 1907, were appointed, one to the East and the other to the West Surgical Service. In 1913, Catherine Conrick, class of 1913, was assigned to the West Surgical Service, having served as an etherizer on the accident service.

In March 1911, Perkins published an article in the first issue of the MGH Nurses' Alumnae Association *Quarterly Record* titled "The Method of Administering, and Various Forms of Anaesthesia in Use, at the Massachusetts General Hospital." In it she reported, "During the past two years I have anesthetized in the vicinity of 1,800 patients at the MGH without serious mishap at the time of operation."

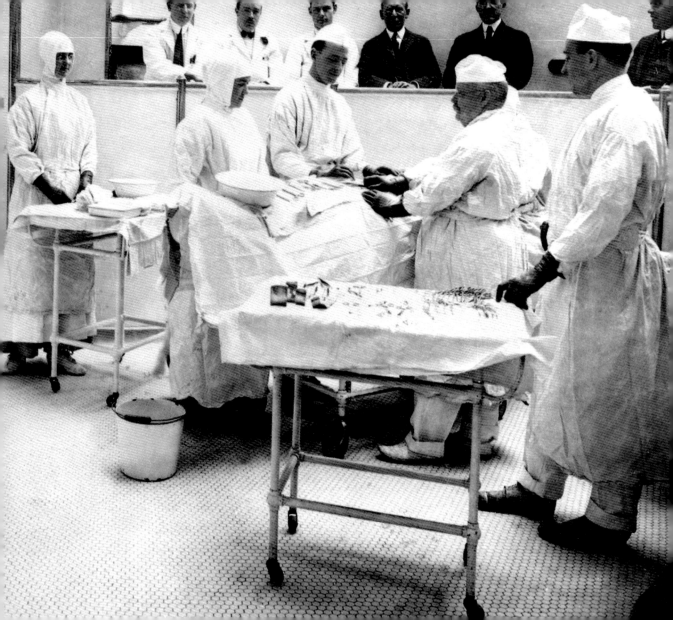

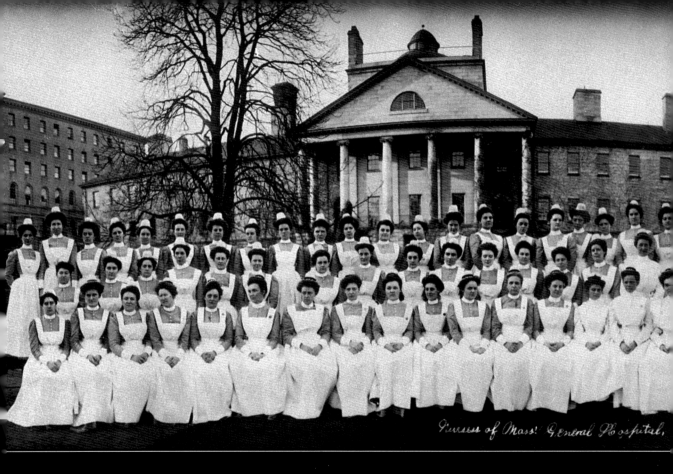

Nurses of Mass! General Hospital.

Pictured is the MGH Nursing staff in 1909. At the time, with the exception of its head nurses, all of the nurses at the hospital were students. It was not until 1925 that the hospital officially hired its first trained staff nurse.

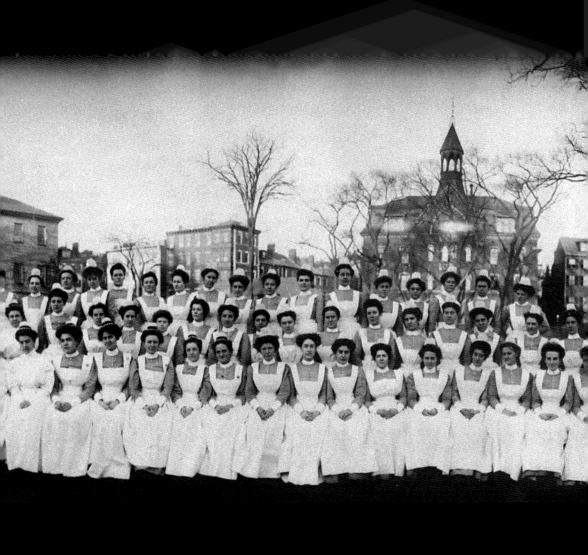

term in the manner of the original appointment. Any
member of the said board may be removed, for cause, by
the governor with the advice and consent of the council.

AN ACT TO PROVIDE FOR THE REGISTRATION OF NURSES.   *Chap.*449

Be it enacted, etc., as follows:

SECTION 1. A Board of Registration of Nurses is
hereby established to consist of five members. One member shall be the secretary of the board of registration in
medicine, ex officio; the other four members shall, within
sixty days after the passage of this act, be appointed by
the governor with the advice and consent of the council.
Three members shall be nurses holding diplomas, each from
a different training school for nurses giving at least a two
years' course in the theory and practice of nursing in a
hospital, and they shall have had eight years' experience
in nursing the sick. The fifth member shall be a physician
who is superintendent of a hospital having a training school
for nurses. The four appointive members shall be appointed to serve as follows: one member for one year,
one for two years, one for three years and one for four
years from the first day of October, nineteen hundred and
ten, and until their respective successors are appointed;
and thereafter the governor, with the advice and consent of
the council, shall annually, before the first day of October,
appoint one person qualified as aforesaid to hold office for
four years from the first day of October next ensuing.
Vacancies in said board shall be filled for the unexpired

[marginal notes]
Board of
Registration
of Nurses
established.

Terms of
office of
members.

Vacancies, etc.

Although the United States passed the first Nurse Practice Acts (rules governing the practice of nursing) in 1903, the effort to enact state laws made uneven progress. The movement, led by the state nurses' associations, had support from some hospital administrators and members of the medical profession, but was opposed by others.

The purpose of state laws was to raise standards in nursing and to protect the public from the untrained or semitrained who called themselves nurses. The state acts established procedures for the registration of nurses under the supervision of a board of nurse examiners. To qualify as a registered nurse, and have the right to use this title, a candidate was required to be a graduate of a training school approved by a state board and to pass a state examination.

The efficiency of the Nurse Practice Acts varied from state to state, as did the effectiveness of the different boards, which prepared and administered the examination and set minimum requirements for the length and content of school training. The Massachusetts Board of Registration in Nursing was established in 1910. Minimum standards were created by 1920, and it is probable that few of the MGH students who encountered an eight-hour "course" in sanitation, or who had to make up days lost through illness or other cause, were aware that these were requirements of some official body of the Commonwealth of Massachusetts.

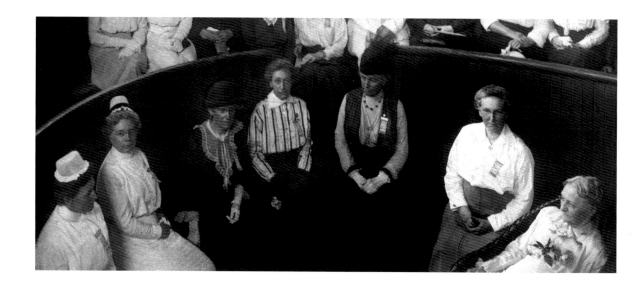

On September 13 and 14, 1915, the Massachusetts General Hospital Nurses' Alumnae Association held its first reunion and produced an impressive gathering of early nurse leaders. Seated in the front row left to right are Annabella McCrae, the school's first full-time instructor, a position she held for 33 years; Sara E. Parsons, superintendent of the Training School, 1910-1920; Pauline L. Dolliver, superintendent, 1899-1909; Carrie M. Hall, superintendent of Nursing, Peter Bent Brigham Hospital; Anna C. Maxwell, superintendent, 1881-1889; Sophia F. Palmer, founder and editor-in-chief, *American Journal of Nursing*, 1900-1920; and Linda Richards, the country's first trained nurse and superintendent of the Training School from 1874 to 1876.

Mary E.P. Davis, class of 1878, was a member of the founding committee (1893) that formed the American Society of Superintendents of Training Schools for Nurses (later known as the National League of Nursing Education), the first national organization for nurses in America. In 1900, she was cofounder and the first business manager of the *American Journal of Nursing*. Miss Davis was a charter member of the American Nurses Association and the third president of the National League of Nursing Education. She served as superintendent of the University of Pennsylvania Hospital Training School, where she organized the first three-year course in nursing. Miss Davis also organized the Central Directory for Nurses in Philadelphia and Boston and was the first registrar of each.

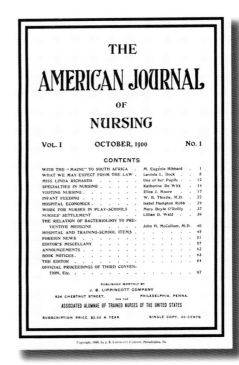

Sophia F. Palmer, class of 1878, was cofounder with Miss Davis of the MGH Nurses' Alumnae Association in 1895. She was the first president of the New York State Board of Nurse Examiners. In 1900, she cofounded and became the first editor of the *American Journal of Nursing*. Miss Palmer was a member of the committees that organized the American Nurses Association and the National League of Nursing Education. She served as superintendent of St. Luke's Hospital in New Bedford, Mass., and then the Rochester Hospital in New York, where the term "registered nurse" was coined. She organized the training school at Garfield Hospital in Washington, D.C. Also of note, she was the first trained nurse to cross the Rocky Mountains in a professional capacity.

As graduates of only the third nursing school in America to be associated with a general hospital, MGH nurses were uniquely positioned to advance their emerging profession. They were among the country's earliest and best trained nurses. Many went on to make significant contributions to nursing during their careers. The following are some of the most prominent early graduates:

Elizabeth Scovil Robinson, class of 1880, authored 21 published books and several articles on nursing and religious subjects. She served as associate editor of the *Ladies Home Journal* for 12 years and on the editorial staff of the *American Journal of Nursing* for 20. She was superintendent of Newport Hospital in Rhode Island from 1888 to 1894.

Annabella McCrae, class of 1895, was a gifted teacher and the first full-time instructor in Nursing Arts in the MGH Training School for Nurses (1912-1935). She was an organizer of the Massachusetts State Nurses Association and the author of *Procedures in Nursing* (1923), which standardized nursing procedures for the first time. She was the inspiration for the phrase "stern teacher, kindly too withal" in the MGH school song.

Garnet I. Pelton, class of 1903, was a pioneer in social work. A graduate of Wellesley College with two years of medical training at Johns Hopkins,

Miss Pelton, in collaboration with Dr. Richard Cabot, organized the first hospital-based Social Service Department in the nation at MGH in 1905. Dr. Cabot noted that "Miss Pelton was, in many ways, the best social worker I have ever seen." That same year she initiated a system of district nursing at Denison House, a neighborhood settlement house in Boston. She later served as first secretary of the Denver Tuberculosis Society and executive secretary of the Colorado Tuberculosis Association.

Harriet L.P. Friend, class of 1904, received her BS and MA from the Teachers College at Columbia and spent her career in nursing education and administration, serving as director of Nursing Education at Temple University in Philadelphia; dean of Knapp College of Nursing in Santa Barbara, Calif., secretary and education director of the Missouri State Board of Nurse Examiners;

director at the headquarters of the California State Nurses' Association; and editor of the *Pacific Coast Journal of Nursing.*

Carrie M. Hall, class of 1904, was the first superintendent of nursing and principal of the nurses' training school at Peter Bent Brigham Hospital from 1912 to 1937. During her tenure, she also served as president of the Massachusetts State Nurses Association (1921-1925) and then as president of the National League for Nursing Education (1926-1928). During World War I, Miss Hall was chief nurse of Base Hospital No. 5 in France, as well as chief nurse of the American Red Cross in Great Britain and France.

Helen Wood, class of 1909, was a 1904 Phi Beta Kappa graduate of Mount Holyoke College and received her master's from the Teachers College at Columbia. She was acting superintendent of Nurses at MGH while Miss Sara E. Parsons served in France (1916-1919). In 1918, a nursing program was arranged with Simmons College, the first college or university connection established with a training school in New England. Miss Wood later became superintendent of nurses at Washington University in St. Louis, Mo. (1919-1923), director of the School of Nursing at the University of Rochester in New York (1924-1931) and director of Nursing at Simmons College in Boston (1933-1946).

Eva S. Waldron, class of 1911, began her nursing career as an operating room nurse at MGH, and then moved on to serve as director of Nursing in Fall River, Mass. With the onset of World War I, she joined the Harvard Medical Unit and eventually was appointed assistant to chief nurse Sara E. Parsons at Base Hospital No. 6 in France. After the war, she returned to Boston and enrolled in Simmons College, earning a certificate in public health. She was a public health nurse in Dover, N.H., for four years before returning to Boston as head of the South End Health Unit, directing care for Boston's ethnic communities and mentoring many young public health nurses. From 1929 to 1954, she was director of the Visiting Nurse Association of Springfield, Mass.

Elizabeth Sullivan, class of 1913, became superintendent of Children's Hospital in Boston and was the first supervisor of Schools of Nursing at the Board of Registration in Nursing in Boston.

Margaret Dieter, class of 1916, was a Phi Beta Kappa graduate of Smith College, and received her master's from the Teachers College at Columbia. She was a missionary in China for five years and then served as director of the School of Nursing at Massachusetts Memorial Hospital from 1926 to 1946. She was president of the Massachusetts State Nurses Association and the Massachusetts League of Nursing and is the author of the MGH school song.

Helen Dore Boylston, class of 1917, served with the Harvard Medical Unit in France during World War I. She is probably best known as the author of the Sue Barton books, which were published between 1936 and 1952 and were thought to be responsible for influencing young women to enter nursing.

Hazel Goff, class of 1917, served in the Army Nurse Corps during World War I and became director of the School of Nursing of the Bulgarian Red Cross in Sophia, Bulgaria. She was also field director of Nursing Service for the Rockefeller Foundation in Paris, France; nurse advisor to the League of Nursing in Geneva; and director of the Red Crescent School, Istanbul, Turkey.

R. Louise Metcalfe, class of 1920, received her BS, MA and PhD from Columbia and initiated the first organized unit to conduct research at the Institute of Research and Nursing at Columbia University. She served as chair of the Florence Nightingale International Council of Nursing, and as professor and chair of the Department of Nursing Education at Columbia, and initiated and established the testing programs of the National League of Nursing Education.

Katherine E. Faville, class of 1921, was the first dean of the Department of Nursing at Wayne State University in Detroit, Mich. Under her leadership, faculty assumed full responsibility for teaching clinical nursing courses, marking the first time clinical teaching shifted from hospital staff to nursing faculty. The Katherine E. Faville Professorship of Nursing Research exists in the College of Nursing at Wayne State University to this day.

Sara E. Parsons, class of 1893, served as superintendent of nurses at the MGH Training School for Nurses from 1910 to 1920.

After her graduate training at McLean Hospital, she established and directed hospitals for the mentally ill in Providence, R.I., and Baltimore, Md. During the Spanish-American War, she served on the hospital ship *Bay State* and in Puerto Rico with Frederic Washburn, MD, director of the General Hospital.

During her tenure as superintendent, Miss Parsons made significant contributions to the school and to nursing and nursing education in general. She faced the challenge of increasing enrollment to meet the hospital's demand for trained nurses while instituting curriculum changes to improve educational standards in nursing education. She initiated surgical bedside clinics and appointed the first full-time instructors in theory applied to nursing and in clinical nursing arts. Miss Parsons advocated for improved working conditions for nurses and enhancements to student nurse life. Recognizing the need to provide scholarships to attract highly qualified candidates, she initiated an endowment fund for the Training School, which continues to provide financial aid for students at the MGH Institute of Health Professions School of Nursing.

In 1916, she took a leave from her superintendent role to prepare an MGH unit for possible service overseas. From 1917 to 1919 — during World War I — she served as chief nurse of Base Hospital No. 6 in France, returning in 1919 to her position as superintendent.

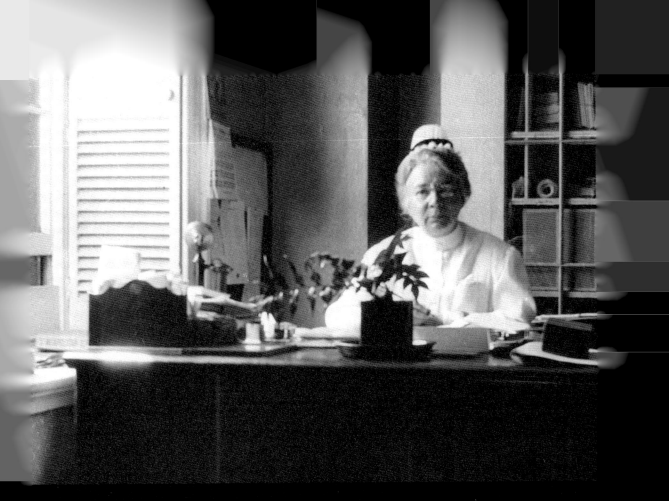

Pictured in her office in 1916, Sara E. Parsons, superintendent of nurses, MGH Training School for Nurses, 1910-1920

oth during and after her career, she as active in nursing alumnae, state nd national organizations, serving s president of the Massachusetts ate Nurses Association and of

Education. She also authored the *History of the MGH Training School for Nurses* (1922) and *Nursing Problems and Obligations* (1928), which became standard for the profession.

When the United States entered World War I in 1917, many changes took place in the routines of both the MGH and the school. The organization of a wartime medical and nursing unit from MGH had begun in 1916. Early in the summer of 1917, the unit sailed for France, and in July it was established near Bordeaux as Base Hospital No. 6. Under the medical direction of Col. Frederic Washburn, the unit included more than 60 nurses, most of them graduates of the hospital's School of Nursing. Sara E. Parsons served as chief nurse.

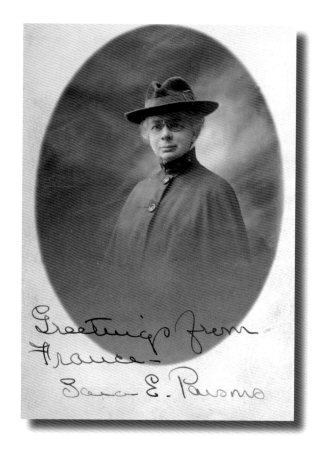

Greetings from France —
Sara E. Parsons

"Most gratifying of all was the spirit of motherliness which pervaded the atmosphere, and the respect which the nurses always commanded."

— Sara E. Parsons, class of 1893,
"The Nurses' Point of View,"
The History of Base Hospital No. 6

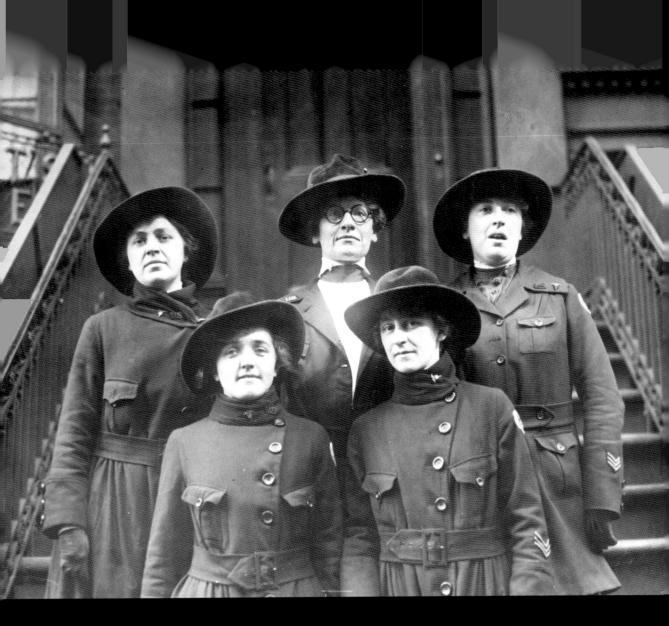

Pictured is a group of Massachusetts General nurses who were among the first American nurses sent to the front with a surgical unit. (l. to r.) TOP ROW: Miss Mary Matheson, Provincetown, Mass.; Miss Helen Nivison, Gardiner, Maine; and Miss Catherine Conrick, Boston; BOTTOM ROW: Miss Glee Marshall, Colbrook, N.H.; and Miss Anna Robertson, Montreal.

In total, more than 200 MGH nurses served overseas during the war, supplying teams of medical personnel for evacuation hospitals, trains, mobile surgical units, and Army camps that received ill and wounded men who required extended treatment.

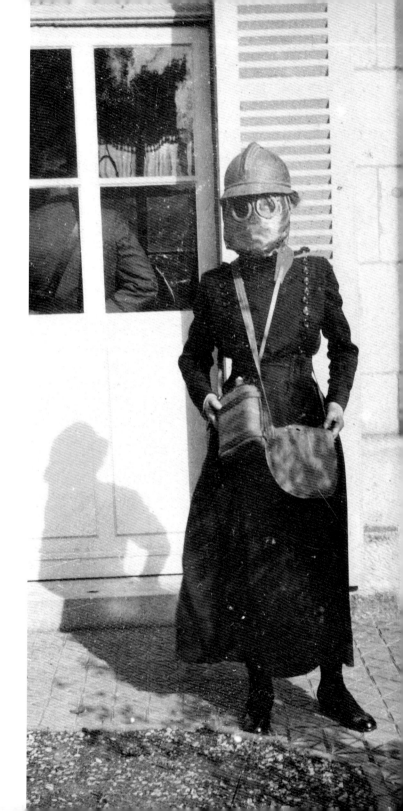

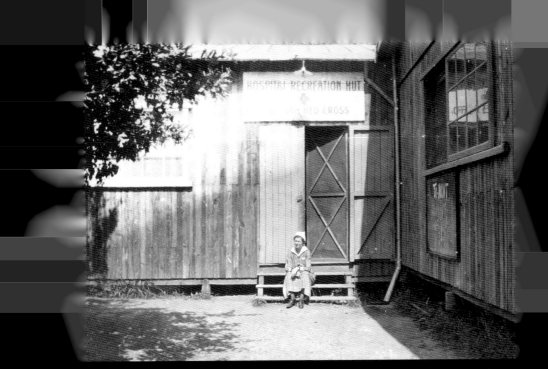

*From Eva Waldron's scrapbook of her time in France
at Base Hospital No. 6 as Sara Parsons' assistant*

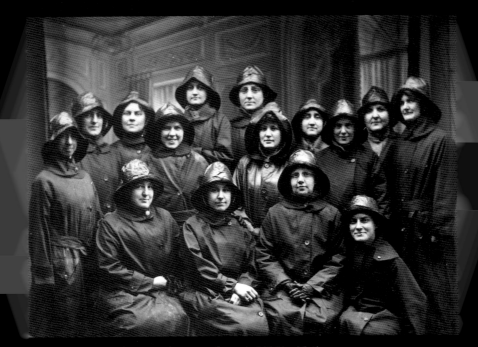

*A postcard was sent home to MGH with the message:
"A Merry Xmas and Happy New Year from the fifteen of Base #13"*

On the morning of December 6, 1917, one of the most devastating events of the 20th century occurred in Halifax, the capital of the Canadian province of Nova Scotia. World War I was into its third year when two European ships from allied countries collided — one loaded with explosives, and the other carrying relief supplies back to Europe. Every house in the city of 50,000 was damaged, some 2,000 people were killed, more than 10,000 were injured — 300 fully or partially blinded — and thousands were left homeless.

Within 24 hours of the disaster, a train loaded with supplies and emergency personnel was making its way from Boston to Nova Scotia. The first relief trains carried members of the Massachusetts State Guard, the Red Cross, and MGH social workers Ruth Emerson and Edith Baker, who helped secure clothing and shelter, arranged special care for injured children, conducted a census of injured persons, and provided psychological assistance. Emerson stayed on in Halifax to help establish the field of medical social service there.

Other first responders who took charge included graduates of the MGH Training School for Nurses: Elizabeth Peden (1899), who was in charge of nurses and supplies for the State Guard Train; Edith I. Cox (1909), who led a Red Cross unit of more than 70 nurses; Edna Harrison (1910); Corine Samuelson (1913); Frances Daily (1907); and Adele Richardson (1915). They spent their first night in Halifax sleeping on the unheated train without food or water, and then — within 24 hours — helped transform the St. Mary's School for Boys into a 150-bed hospital containing separate wards for women, men and children; an operating room for minor surgery; an outpatient department; and the usual administrative necessities of any hospital.

In gratitude, Halifax gave the people of Boston a Christmas tree in December 1918, and in 1971 that city made the Christmas tree gift an annual tradition.

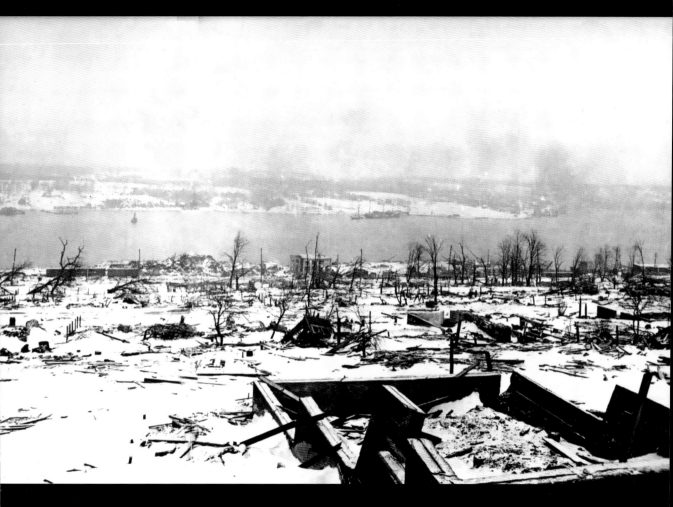

The aftermath of the 1917 Halifax explosion that left 2,000 people dead, more than 10,000 injured and thousands homeless

"As leaders and staff among medical and nursing groups departed overseas, there was considerable disruption. ... New and inexperienced workers had to be absorbed, and there were never enough. ... The ones who remained at home had quite as difficult a task."

When the armistice came on November 11, 1918, Base Hospital No. 6 had treated more than 4,300 patients. The unit returned home in February 1919.

The chief problem, steadily increasing even before World War I, was the demand for more and more service from the nurses (students) as the doctors introduced new procedures and conducted research.

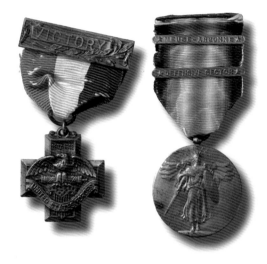

Following the war, the town of Claremont, N.H., awarded the above medal inscribed "Victory" (above left) to Lillian Augusta Osgood, RN, class of 1917. The back features the town seal and the inscription "Presented by the Town of Claremont, N.H., in recognition of patriotic services in the World War." She also received a U.S. "Victory Medal" (above right) with a "Defensive Sector" service clasp on the ribbon. The reverse is inscribed "The Great War for Civilization" and features an American shield and list of the Allied and Associated nations.

NEW ENGLAND HEROINES BACK FROM THE FRONT

Massachusetts General Hospital Unit Arrives in New York— 69 Nurses and 25 Surgeons—Were Under Fire Sharing Dangers of the 26th and Other U. S. Divisions

Work of Mercy Extended Over Period of 20 Months— Get Great Welcome

Thrilling Stories Told of the Bravery of Women Who Knew No Fear

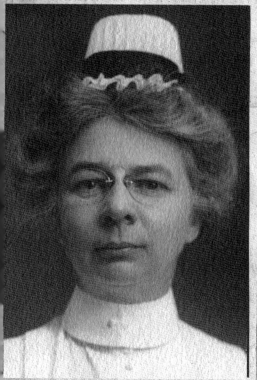

MISS SARA E. PARSONS,
uperintendent of nurses of the Massachusetts General Hospital, and head nurse of the Massachusetts General Hospital Unit, which returned from France yesterday. Miss Parsons declared that the nurses who served under her direction "did not know what fear meant."

BY HAROLD F. WHEELER
Post Staff Correspondent

NEW YORK, March 2.—Sixty-nine world war heroines came into this city tonight bringing stories that must live always to the honor and glory of Boston and New England.

Nurses these heroines, nurses of the Massachusetts General Hospital Unit of Boston, who made up Base Hospital No. 6 of the American expeditionary forces in France.

All had seen 20 months' service— wore three gold service stripes on the left sleeves of their blue army nurses' uniforms—and all had run the gamut of war's hell.

There were those among them who had spent weeks at a time—months, even — just behind the front line trenches; were under fire with the 26th, Boston and New England's own Yankee Division, at Seicheprey, at Argonne, at St. Mihiel, at Verdun; were under fire with other divisions at other

Eighty Nurses Graduated in Victory Class at Mass. General Hospital

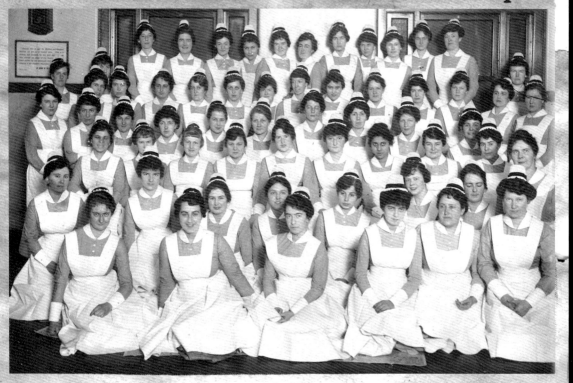

GRADUATING CLASS OF 1919 OF THE MASSACHUSETTS GENERAL HOSPITAL.
Photo by Harry J. Kelly.

"Eighty young women, constituting the 'Victory' class of the Massachusetts General Hospital, after completing the hardest year of continuous hard nursing that has ever been done by pupil nurses in the history of the institution, were graduated last night. Dr. Henry P. Walcott, chairman of the board of trustees, who presided at the exercises and announced the graduates, declared that each individual member of the class had done as high a service and incurred as grave a danger as any nurse or soldier in service abroad." Article from the scrapbook of Jane Austin Sullivan, RN, class of 1919, back row, third from the left.

— Above and right from The Trained Nurse and Hospital Review, *1919*

While many overseas faced great danger in 1918, those at home were also at risk. One of the greatest pandemics ever to hit Boston occurred. It has been estimated that between September 1, 1918, and January 16, 1919, approximately 45,000 people died from influenza in Massachusetts alone. An unidentified newspaper article that accompanied the photograph at left describes the impact on nursing at MGH, in particular:

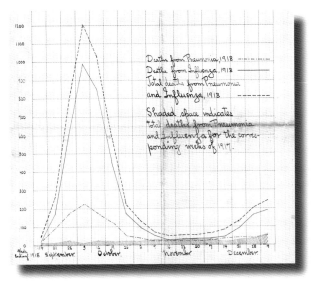

According to an inscription on the reverse, the above "Boston Influenza Chart" accompanied a January 12, 1919, article in the Sunday News. *It compares the deaths from pneumonia and influenza in Boston during September and October of 1917 and 1918. Courtesy of the Boston Public Library.*

800 CASES OF FLU

"The members of the class have in the past year nursed over 800 cases of influenza which came in two great waves. Over half of the class were seriously ill with the disease; and all, because of the severe tax which overwork placed upon them, were made dangerously susceptible. One of their number died. A scarlet fever epidemic placed 36 of the girls on the dangerous list, but all survived.

"'There are no words,' said Dr. Henry Van Dyke, who made the address of the evening, 'that can fittingly commend the part that women, and especially nurses, have played in the winning of the war. The type of service that did not flinch even before an enemy that chose as its favorite target that Red Cross on the roof of a hospital, can never be given its just reward in rhetoric.'"

A Song for M.G.H.

Words by M. Dieter   M.S.W.

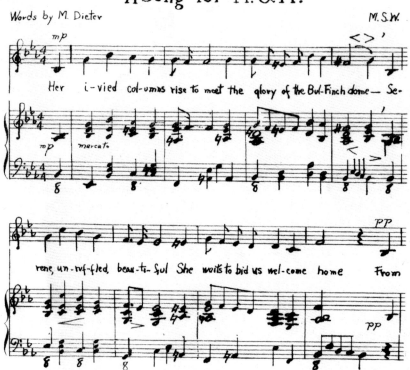

1.

Her ivied columns rise to meet
the glory of the Bulfinch dome
Serene, unruffled, beautiful
She waits to bid us welcome home.

From many lands, o're many days
We brought to her our restless youth.
And she with patience took us all
And set us on the way to truth.

2.

Stern Teacher, kindly too, withal
Who saw the faults we could not hide.
And building on our better selves,
She wrought results that shall abide.

What if she gave us arduous toil,
She taught us reverence for our work,
To ease the suffering, lighten pain,
There is no task we dare to shirk.

Song for MGH, by Margaret Dieter, class of 1916. While Miss Sara Parsons was serving in France, Miss Dieter sent her a Christmas card enclosing a poem she had written. This was later set to music and became the school song, first sung at graduation in 1922 and at all functions into the 1960s. In 2010, the Nursing Alumnae Association added the fourth verse, written by its president-elect, Vareen O'Keefe-Domaleski, RN, EdD, class of 1971.

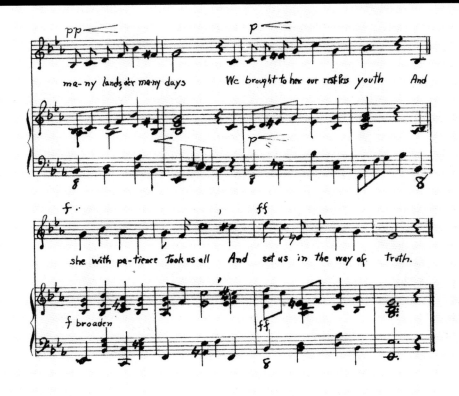

3.	4
Where life and death are side by side,	A century and more has passed
And creeds and races strangely blend,	Our legacy alive and strong
To share these things from day to day	Our lives touch those around the globe
She helped us each to find a friend.	And with great pride we sing this song.
Oh, Gracious Guardian of our past,	The world has changed and so must we,
Thy children rise to honor thee.	Yet values keep our actions true
God bless and keep you, MGH,	The gift of caring for the sick
Secure through all the years to be.	Transforms their lives and our lives too.

93

Ward Rules for Nurses

WARDS should be in order by 10 A.M. Each nurse must give her own medicines, except those given by the medicine-week nurse. She must serve her own patients' meals; carry back and scrape her own dishes; wash all utensils she uses between meals; keep her beds in order; sweep her own side of the ward; dust every day; and keep her bedside stands and fruit-closet shelves clean. She is expected to take up her share of another nurse's work conscientiously when that nurse is off the ward.

Dishes, fruit, clothes, etc., must not be left on stands or on window-sills. If toilet paper is left in the stand drawers, the sheets must be fastened with a safety pin. In male wards urinals must be kept on the lower shelves of the bedside tables. They must be promptly emptied; patients should be instructed to request that this be done.

Patients who are in bed all day should have their beds freed from crumbs after each meal.

At night beds must be straightened and clothes tightened; the stands must be cleared of books, papers, and the like; wrappers must be hung in the lockers; and backs rubbed with bathing solution.

Children and all patients who have special nurses should be bathed daily. With these exceptions, women patients should be bathed every

When in Doubt Consult the Supervisor

3

A chronic issue in nursing was the confusion and uncertainty over the nurse's duties and responsibilities. Nurses were frequently employed in work for which they were not trained, and they were often far from sources of help or supervision. In the absence of a clear understanding of objectives, no one, whether a school administrator, teacher, hospital administrator, Trustee, or medical staff member, really knew whether a course of study for nurses was adequate or not.

An MGH pamphlet titled "Night Nurses, 1919-1920" provided specific direction for the staff and a glimpse of nursing practice at that time.

Excerpts, "Ward Rules for Nurses"

Wards should be in order by 10 a.m. Each nurse must give her own medicines, except those given by the medicine-week nurse. She must serve her own patients' meals; carry back and scrape her own dishes; wash all utensils she uses between meals; keep her beds in order; sweep her own side of the ward; dust every day; and keep her bedside stands and fruit-closet shelves clean. She is expected to take up her share of another nurse's work conscientiously when that nurse is off the ward.

... All orders must be written in the order-book by a house-officer, except at night when verbal orders may be given — these to be written in the order-book by the nurse and initialed by the house-officer on his morning visit. The nurse who carries out the order should cross it off in the book.

... Medicine and fruit closets and clothes lockers must be kept locked.

Visitors

...The visiting hour is from 2 to 3 p.m. Patients over twelve years of age are allowed to have one visitor daily. On Saturdays each patient may be visited by one adult and one child; and on holidays by two adults. For children under twelve the only visiting days are Saturdays and holidays when they are governed by the same rule as adults. This restriction applies to all children under twelve in the hospital, not merely to those in Ward H. A patient on the danger list is usually allowed two visitors at any time. If more than two visitors are present, all in excess of the legitimate number should be sent back to the waiting-room at the front entrance.

Admission of Patient

The nurses are expected to receive new patients with special courtesy and consideration. The temperature, pulse, and respiration must be taken as soon as possible. This is followed by a thorough tub bath, except when the temperature is over 101° he should be put to bed.

After the temperature, pulse, and respiration have been ascertained, the admission with this data must be reported to the proper house-officer. Clothes must be marked and listed in duplicate (one list for the telephone office and one for the ward) and placed in a clothes-locker. So far as possible superfluous and soiled clothing should be returned to the friends who accompany a patient. The patient's hair should be combed with a fine comb, and if pediculi or nits are found, tincture of larkspur must be applied. The body and seams of clothing must also be inspected carefully for body parasites. If these are found the clothes are at once marked and sent "special" to the laundry. ...

Discharge of Patient

His card is taken to the window of the telephone office, then to the admitting physician, then to the cashier, and finally is left on the desk of the admitting physician. No exceptions may be made to this rule when the cashier's office is open. The form on the back of the card must be accurately filled out at the time of discharge. Be sure that the date of discharge is correct. Unless the patient is on a stretcher he should accompany the nurse to the various departments. ...

When a patient has been discharged, the mattresses and pillows are to be marked with ward number and date and sent to the mattress room after having been brushed with 2% formaldehyde. If the mattress has been used for a contagious case, such as erysipelas, the name of the disease must be added to the slip sewed to the mattress. Rubber sheet and the bed shall be washed with corrosive sublimate 1-3000. ...

Laundry

In sorting soiled linen for the laundry care should be taken to eliminate safety pins, rubber sheets, or any other article not properly belonging in the laundry. Mutilated articles should be withdrawn and reported to the head nurse, who in turn should investigate the cause of damage and report the same to the supervisors. Then the articles should be sent in "special" to the head laundress.

The bags should be ready for collection at 10 a.m. and 7 p.m. (on Saturdays at 4 p.m. also). Two receptacles for gauze, compress, and bandages are in each ward. In one receptacle should be put dressing materials from case of (a) Typhoid fever, Erysipelas, Syphilis, Anthrax, Faecal Fistulae, Gauze to which adhesive plaster or hair are attached, and marked "Boiler House."

(b) All other gauze, compress, and bandages must be placed in the second receptacle that they may be saved and washed. At noon and night all dressings must be transferred to paper bags clearly marked with the ward letter or number. Dressings ... to be destroyed are placed in a bag also marked "Boiler House."

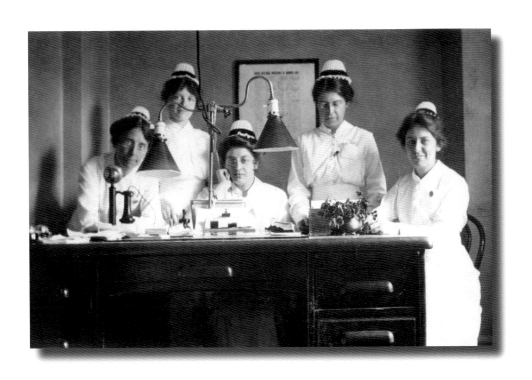

Each afternoon the head nurse must requisition for the necessary supply of linen for use the next day. Double supply must be ordered on Saturdays and the day before a holiday. On each requisition she shall put the number of patients, and if there are any who require an unusual supply, a note shall be made on the requisition to that effect. A reasonable amount of extra linen for emergencies may be asked for.

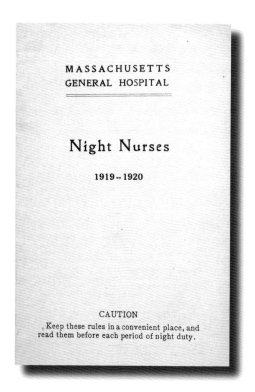

MASSACHUSETTS
GENERAL HOSPITAL

Night Nurses

1919--1920

CAUTION
Keep these rules in a convenient place, and
read them before each period of night duty.

Night Nurses

When on duty night nurses shall remain in the wards to which they are assigned, except when they have to report a case. On such occasion, they shall notify the nurse in the adjoining ward that they are about to leave. Except in an emergency, they shall report to the night superintendent of nurses before they call a house-officer. No officer or employee is allowed to obtain lunch in a ward.

Night nurses are required to set the trays for breakfast; turn on steam in steam table; wash all dishes used during the night; leave sinks and bathrooms in order; prepare soiled clothes for the laundry; report anything loaned, borrowed, or broken; see that all patients are washed and have their teeth brushed before breakfast; make beds as directed; report at meals not later than 7:15 a.m. or 6 p.m.

GENERAL RULES
for
NIGHT NURSES
1919 - 1920

"Special responsibility rests on the evening nurse and on the night nurse, as they alone must maintain order and quiet in the wards as well as care properly for the patients.

Give particular attention to new patients and observe them closely. Understand as far as possible the condition and disease of each patient. See each patient at least every twenty minutes. Any medication or work which will confine you to one patient for more than half an hour should be reported to the Night Supervisor who will secure help if possible.

Report at once to Night Supervisor when a bed patient falls or gets out of bed."

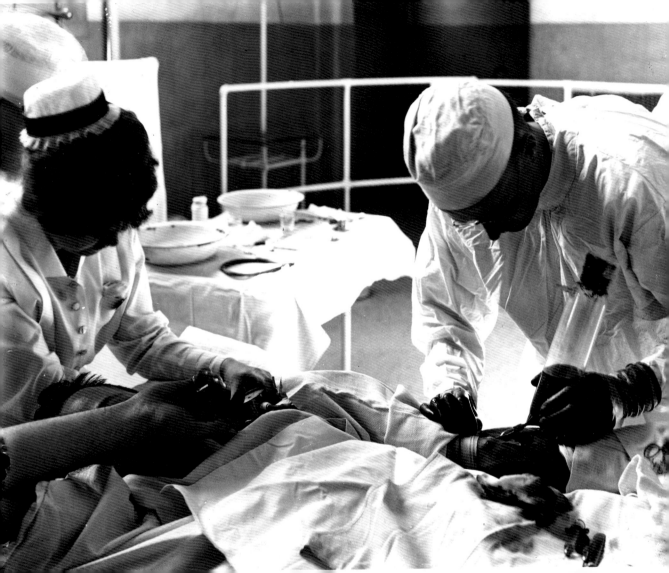

Conscientious nursing often prevented complications for both medical and surgical patients. In the early 1900s, before the days of early ambulation, nursing was particularly important because patients were more vulnerable to pneumonia and the necrosis of tissues over bony prominences, such as knees or elbows. Mouth care, back care, turning from side to side, and other positioning were crucial not only to the patient's comfort but even to life. With antibiotics as yet unknown, the nurse carried a heavy responsibility, and often played a part at least equal to that of the doctor.

The good private-duty nurse was indeed the doctor's right hand, and in the long hours between his visits, she was his eyes and ears as well. Multiple changes that soon appeared in medicine did much to challenge this relationship between the nurse and the doctor. The doctor of the 1920s in many ways stood halfway between the largely empirical practices of the past and a new, scientifically based care of patients.

In 1925, the MGH opened the second clinical research center in the United States, a 10-bed unit in the Bulfinch Building, known as Ward 4 and later renamed the Mallinckrodt General Clinical Research Center. The criteria for admitting patients to Ward 4 was that its special facilities be required to accomplish certain studies that competent investigators, with the patient's cooperation, wished to undertake. The unit was specifically designed to foster clinical research in medicine. The ward's professional staff, who devoted their full attention to its affairs, were the head nurses and the dietitians.

Their devotion was credited with making the success of the ward possible. They "have kept the ward going smoothly and always ready to serve the cause of research, yet at the same time they have seen that the nursing and dietetic care of all patients in the ward is constantly of first-class quality. The head nurse has a great deal to do with setting the tone of the ward and with holding it together as a cooperative unit. She indoctrinates patients in the cause of research and their own contribution to it. Above all, she takes the lead in promoting their happiness during their stay in the ward. Always a graduate nurse herself, the head nurse usually had four pupil nurses to help her carry out her many duties."

Over the years the Mallinckrodt Unit continued to conduct clinical research with nurses as part of the team. As the hospital increased the scope of scientific and medical research, physicians sought and were granted funds for their research. Many of these grants included money to hire staff and nurses who were specifically interested in clinical research.

Nurses' early work in research was usually hidden behind their exceptional ability to improvise and invent while using the everyday equipment of patient care, such as bedside tables, thermometers and stethoscopes. Behind their use of this developing science and technology was their unflagging commitment to the relationship that they had with their patients, which is the foundation of the current state of nursing research and science.

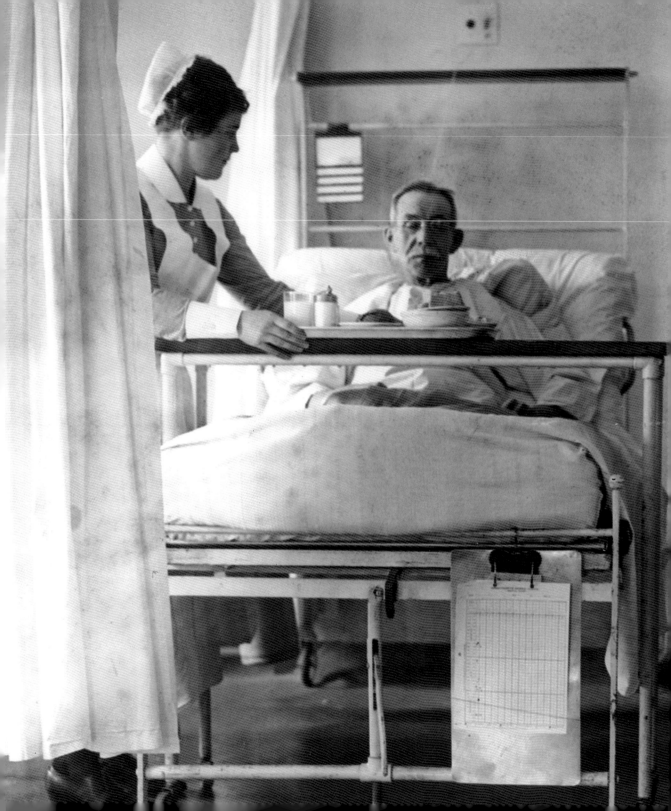

In the early years, only a few states required that a registered nurse be a high school graduate, and neither New York nor Massachusetts were among them. The 1925 revision of the New York Syllabus, containing the law and a sample curriculum to be used as a guide, specified that the candidate for state registration must have a "preliminary education of not less than one year of high school or its equivalent, such educational requirement not to be increased before the year 1930." New York achieved the high school diploma requirement in 1932. Massachusetts required a minimum of one year of high school before 1922, when two years were specified; the high school diploma became a requirement in 1934. This comparison shows not only the relatively high standards that had been achieved at the MGH but also the prevalent practice of scheduling half or more of a student's class work in her first four months.

At right, a summary curriculum from the 1921-1922 Massachusetts General Hospital Training School for Nurses

MASSACHUSETTS GENERAL HOSPITAL

CURRICULUM, 1921–22

SUMMARY

SUBJECTS	LECTURES AND CLASSES	LAB.	TOTAL HOURS	POINTS	INSTRUCTOR
PRELIMINARY COURSE					
Anatomy and Physiology .	55	25	80	4	Nurse Inst.
Chemistry	12	12	24	1	Nurse Inst.
Bacteriology . . .	15	15	30	1 ½	Nurse Inst.
Drugs and Solutions . .	5	10	15	½	Nurse Inst.
Social Service . . .	8		8	½	Soc. Serv. Worker
Dietetics and Cookery .	16	32	48	2	Dietitian
History of Nursing and Ethics	16		16	1	Supt. of Nurses
Practical Nursing					
Demonstrations . . .	90				
Practice in classroom .		90			
Supervised practice on ward		204			
Total of practical nursing			384	12	Nurse Inst.
JUNIOR YEAR (last half of first year)					
Materia Medica . . .	20		20	1	Nurse Inst.
Bandaging and First Aid .	6	8	14	½	Surgeon and Nurse Inst.
Medical Nursing, 1st half .	24	8	32	credited below	Physician and Nurse Inst.
INTERMEDIATE YEAR					
Medical Nursing, 2d half .	24	8	32	3 ½	Phys. and Nurse Inst.
Massage	4	8	12	1	Masseuse
Sanitation	8		8	½	Phys. and Inst.
Urinalysis	1	1	2		Phys. and Inst.
Surgical Nursing . . .	32	32	64	3 ½	Surgeons and Nurse Inst.
SENIOR YEAR					
Obstetrical Nursing . .	30	15	45	2 ½	Obstetricians and Nurse Inst.
Nursing and Its History, Problems and Opportunities . . .	30		30	2	Supt. of Nurses
Special Lectures . . .	30		30	2	Specialists
Oral Hygiene . . .					
X-Ray, Radium . . .					
Tuberculosis . . .					
Syphilis					
Diseases of Eye, Ear, Nose and Throat . .					
Skin Diseases . . .					
Nutrition					
Serum Therapy . . .					
Occupational Therapy .					
Social Hygiene . . .					
Hospital Administration					
Ethics					
	426	468	894	39	

All doctors took it for granted that nursing students would care for patients everywhere except in the private Phillips House, and that the head nurses and students would assist the medical and surgical staffs in various ways. Some doctors regarded the student as a learner seeking an education, to which they contributed generously. Others wanted a helper with some training, but did not expect the trainee to have a basic education. Still others expected the student to have a sound knowledge of biological science and were disconcerted to find, when they needed to explain some test or treatment, that the student nurse could not understand because she lacked the necessary background.

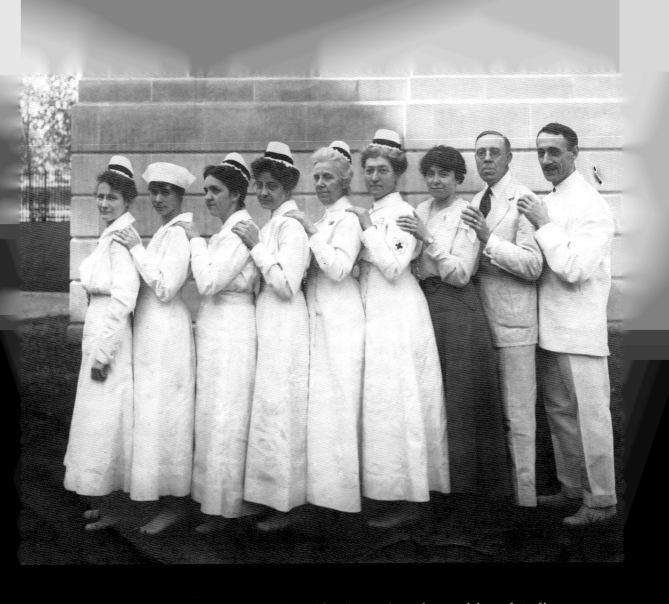

Phillips House was established in 1916 as MGH's ward for private patients who wanted the comforts of home while enjoying the benefits of first-rate medical care. In 2011, it still exists on the top three floors of the Ellison Building. Pictured above is the original Phillips House staff: (l. to r.) Miss Morgan (1916) head nurse, first floor; Miss Harrison, dietician; Miss Alice Barnard (1916), head nurse, OR; Miss Louise Zutter (1913), assistant superintendent; Miss Pauline Dolliver (1889), superintendent; Miss Minnie Hollingsworth (1897), X-ray Department; an unidentified bookkeeper; an unidentified orderly; and Fred Warner, an orderly in the OR.

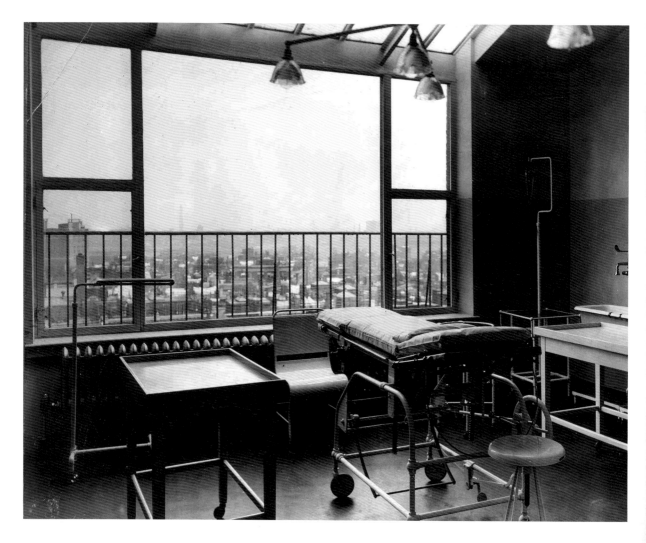

Operating Room in Phillips House as it appeared in 1917

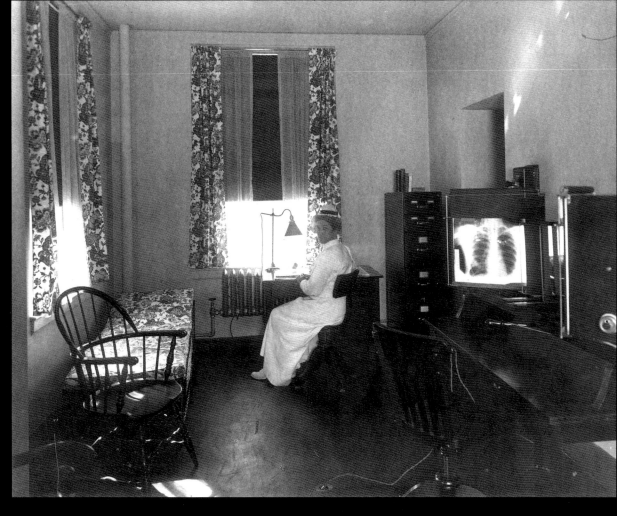

Phillips House X-ray nurse, c. 1920

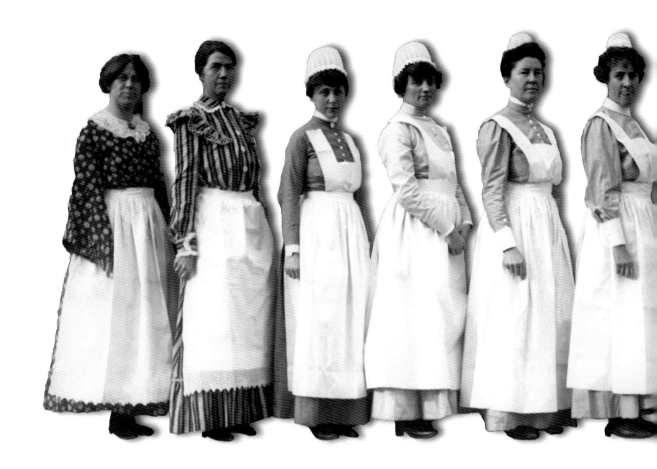

The earliest MGH nurses wore the plain long dresses of the day. Some time around 1874, Linda Richards introduced uniform collars and cuffs. In 1881, one of the lady visitors suggested uniform dress for nurses. For several years, the nurses continued to wear print dresses of an inconspicuous pattern. If a nurse wore a dress of pronounced design, she was threatened with a uniform. In 1884, then-superintendent Miss Maxwell persuaded the school's directors to have a badge made for the school, and she planned a uniform for the pupils: a gingham dress of turquoise blue and white broken check, a gathered apron with bib straps pinned at the shoulder and tied around the waist with bow and strings, and straight collars and cuffs worn inside the neck band and sleeves. The MGH cap was nearly large enough to cover the hair. Because the uniforms

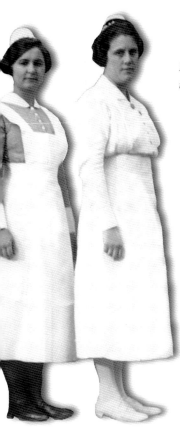

Pictured (left) are MGH nurses in period dress from the early 1800s through the mid-1920s.

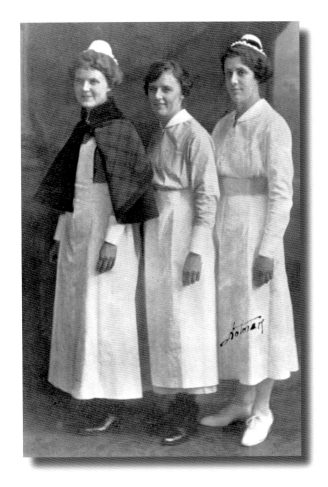

Pictured above are three MGH nurses in 1922 at different points in their careers. The uniforms illustrate their status: (l. to r.) student nurse, preliminary nurse and graduate nurse.

faded when laundered, a black and white checked gingham was introduced, which remained a permanent feature of the uniform. Graduate nurses eventually universally adopted the classic white nursing uniform. As reasoned within a 1906 *American Journal of Nursing* editorial, "A nurse in a sickroom is supposed to wear clean clothing, her uniform of a washable material so that it may be clean and not hold the germs of disease."

View of North Anderson Street looking north to the Bulfinch Building, c. 1928. The MGH's environs were less than prosperous in the 1920s.

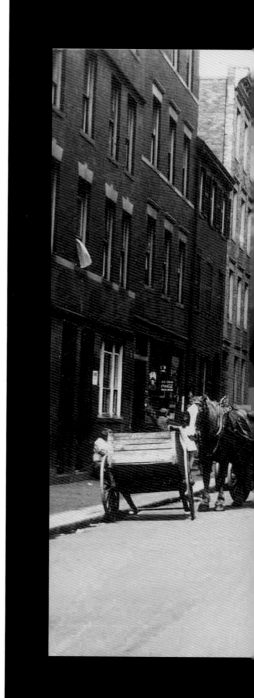

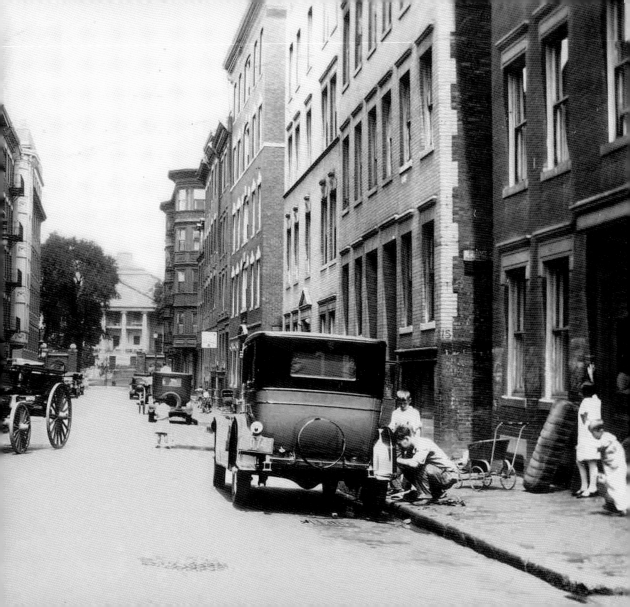

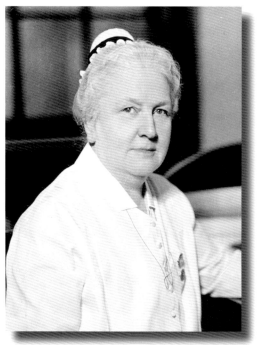

Sally Johnson, RN, class of 1910, served for a quarter-century as superintendent of nurses and principal of the School of Nursing at MGH. When she retired in 1946, the school had 3,060 alumnae, two-thirds of whom had graduated under her.

Miss Johnson began her career teaching fifth grade, which she did for nine years before entering nursing. The values most often attributed to her were loyalty, integrity and responsibility. She was quick to learn and shrewd in sizing up people and situations, but humble in assessing her own abilities.

After graduation she did a postgraduate course at McLean Hospital and then became an instructor of practical nursing at St. Luke's Hospital in New Bedford. In 1912, she became the instructor of practical nursing at the new Peter Bent Brigham Hospital, and in 1913 was appointed assistant superintendent of nurses. In 1917, she became superintendent of nurses and principal of the school of nursing at the Albany Hospital (NY). There she organized the nursing service of the American Red Cross Base Hospital of the Albany Hospital and was chosen to assist in the development of the Army School of Nursing at Walter Reed Hospital in Washington, D.C.

Among her many accomplishments at the MGH, she hired the first floor-duty nurse in the General Hospital in 1924, the first ward secretary in 1929, and she opened a reference library for nurses in 1930.

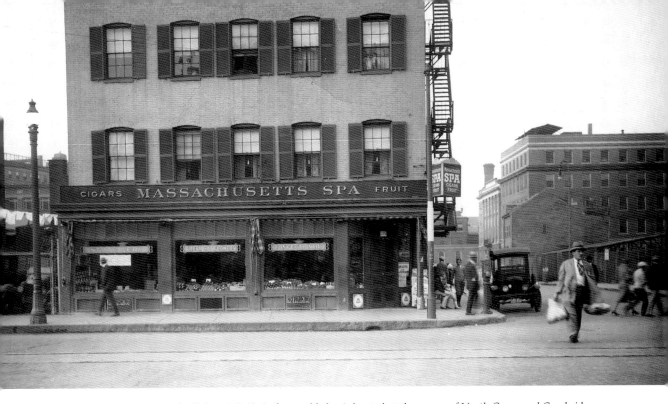

Massachusetts Spa Minichiello's or Mini's (referenced below), located at the corner of North Grove and Cambridge streets, the current location of the Resident Physician's House, c. 1925

Miss Johnson was known for running a tight ship, as exemplified by the following excerpt from one of her famous notices, which were issued regularly and posted widely:

"Under no circumstances are students to use North Anderson, West Cedar, or any other street on the hill when in uniform. Nurses must not appear on the street in uniform, except when going to and from the hospital. The MGH cape is not to be worn on the street in severe weather. Nurses must not stop anywhere on errands between the hospital and the Charles Street Home when in uniform, except Minichiello's [store]. It is expected that nurses will be quiet and dignified and cover the distance between the home and the hospital in as short a time as possible." (Sept. 1932)

In 1930, the Baker Memorial Hospital for People of Moderate Means opened to serve patients who did not qualify for free care but would have difficulty paying the full fees without assistance. A sliding scale enabled such patients to pay what they could afford to the hospital and to their treating physicians.

At the time, there were 109 beds in the Phillips House and 420 in the general hospital wards. The Baker had potential space for 320 patients, its own X-ray equipment, operating rooms, an obstetrical division and dietary service. The typical floor housed 37 patients in single and semiprivate rooms.

With the opening of the Baker, hospital officials hoped to increase the general standard for nursing instead of creating a special nursing service for the building. Fees for Baker patients allowed more graduate nurses to be hired, and a movement to standardize nursing across the wards at MGH began.

One basic element in the Baker plan was to have such high-quality nursing services that the need and expense of special nurses would be eliminated. This meant that in the Baker, at least, the heavy load of nursing care borne by students would be lightened, and better supervision would be given to their work.

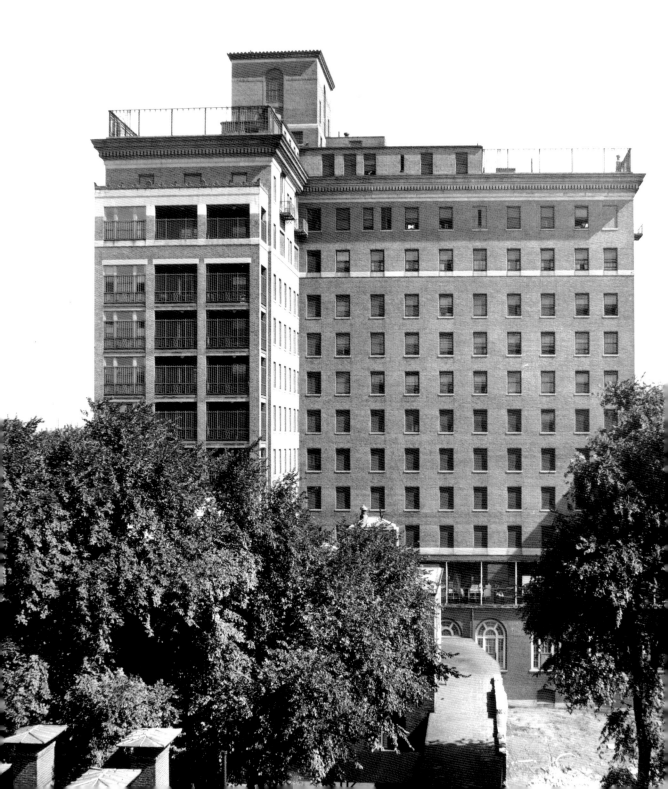

Ruth Sleeper, RN, BS, MA, class of 1922, is widely credited with raising the professional standards for nursing nationwide. Miss Sleeper began her relationship with the MGH as a student in the School of Nursing. From 1933 to 1946, she served as the assistant superintendent of Nursing and assistant principal of the School of Nursing. From 1947 to 1966, she served both as the director of the MGH School of Nursing and the hospital's Nursing Service — a time when nursing was evolving from a hospital-based apprenticeship into a profession requiring academic training and practical experience. Her decision to revise the school's curriculum to reflect this shift was considered revolutionary, yet soon became the standard for nurses' training. She was a firm supporter of academic education and worked to establish affiliations with colleges and universities to ensure that nurses would have a broader academic base and a degree. Even after her retirement she continued to work to transform the MGH School of Nursing into a degree-granting school.

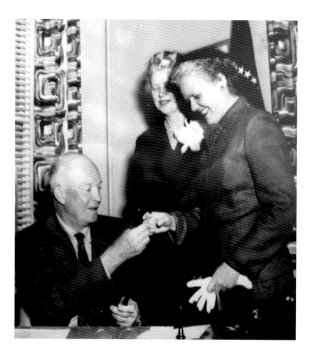

President Eisenhower presents his pen to Ruth Sleeper after he declared National Nurse Week in 1954.

Nationally, Miss Sleeper served as president of the National League of Nursing Education and later as the first president of the National

League for Nursing. Additionally, she was chair of the Nursing Advisory Committee of the Veteran's Administration; member of the National Nursing Council for War Service; member of the Health Resources Advisory Committee, Office of Defense Mobilization, U.S. State Department; Consultant to the U.S. Public Health Division of Nursing Education; and member of the American Red Cross Advisory Board on Health and Human Services, among others.

Miss Sleeper was also well-known and respected internationally. She served as chairman of the Education Committee of the International Council of Nursing (1947-1961), as a member of the Expert Committee on Nursing of the World Health Organization, with the Florence Nightingale International Foundation and as a member of the Commission on the Status of Women at the Meeting of Economic and Social Council of the United Nations.

"Always, always more to see,

more to learn, more to do ...

to improve both care and cure."

— Ruth Sleeper, class of 1922,
director of the MGH School of Nursing
and the MGH Nursing Service

In 1937, Miss Sleeper conducted a study for the reorganization of the MGH School of Nursing. At the time, student nurses comprised the vast majority of the hospital nursing staff. Excerpts from the report describe the tremendous demands placed on their shoulders.

"The student nurse at the MGH carries a disproportionate share of the nursing load. As part of their so-called education, the student nurse gives approximately 85% of the bedside nursing care in the General Hospital, approximately 18% of the bedside nursing care in the Baker Memorial and exclusive of four head nurses, carries out 100% of the nursing care in the clinics of the General Hospital Out-Patient Department. ... Her work week includes 52 hours of ward duty in addition to 4-6 hours of class. After the first four months, except for 3 weeks each year, the typical MGH student never has 24 hours free for her own use."

The report went on to recommend changes to the nursing school curriculum that included requiring the hospital to hire 90 graduate nurses to provide the nursing care that was being provided by MGH student nurses, at a cost to the hospital of $106,758.72.

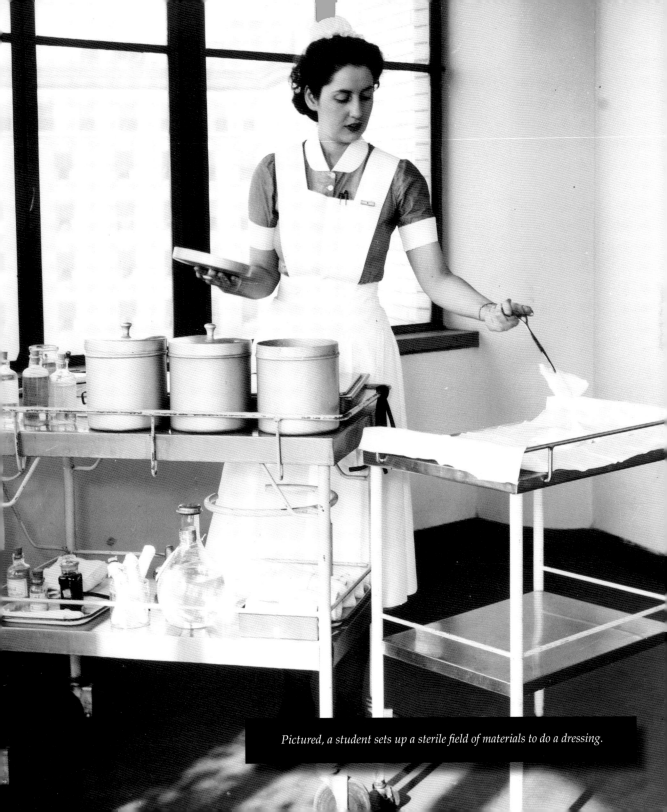

Pictured, a student sets up a sterile field of materials to do a dressing.

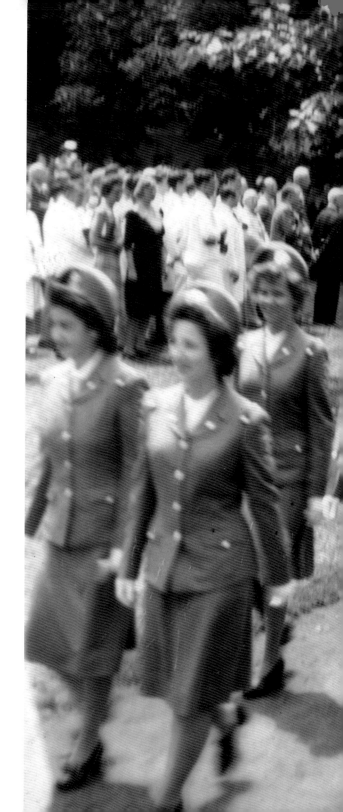

The national Nurse Training Act of 1941 provided $1.2 million to fund student nurses, refresher courses for inactive nurses and postgraduate courses in specialty areas. The Nurse Training Act of 1943 created a $65 million program called the U.S. Cadet Nurse Corps. The Cadet Nurse Corps was terminated by the end of World War II, and by 1949 the last student had graduated. During 1945, 85 percent of nursing students in the country were cadet nurses.

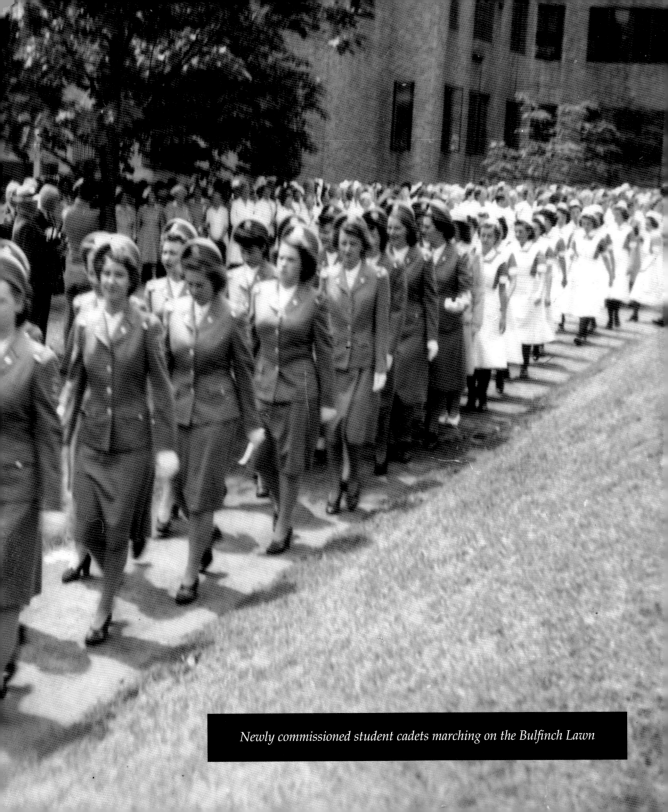

Newly commissioned student cadets marching on the Bulfinch Lawn

Many MGH nurses continued the hospital's tradition of answering the call to service:

"In 1935, I entered Massachusetts General Hospital as a probationer [six months]. Our superintendent of nurses, Sally Johnson, related the history of Mass General, invariably mentioning WWI and Base Hospital No. 6. I couldn't imagine why she kept mentioning this ancient history but came to find out that when WWI ended, Base Hospital No. 6 served as a model for the 6th General Hospital in World War II [a U.S. Army base hospital].

"A reserve unit was established, which was inactive until 1940, the start of WWII. At that time it was clear that it was only a matter of time before the U.S. would be involved.

"In 1940 the War Department asked many academic institutions to set up staffs for active duty. The MGH unit ended up as 40 percent of doctors and 30 percent of nursing staff."

— *Geraldine Brandon Reddington, class of 1938, served at the 6th General Hospital.*

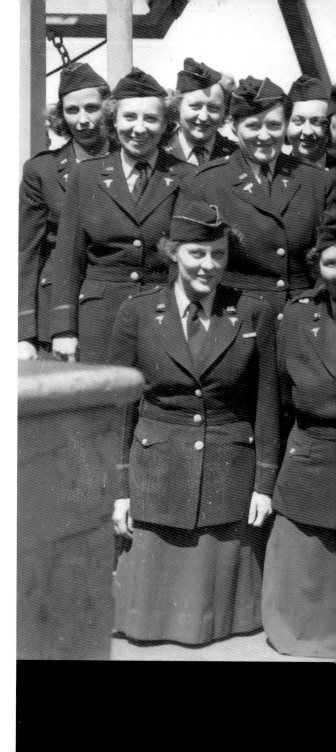

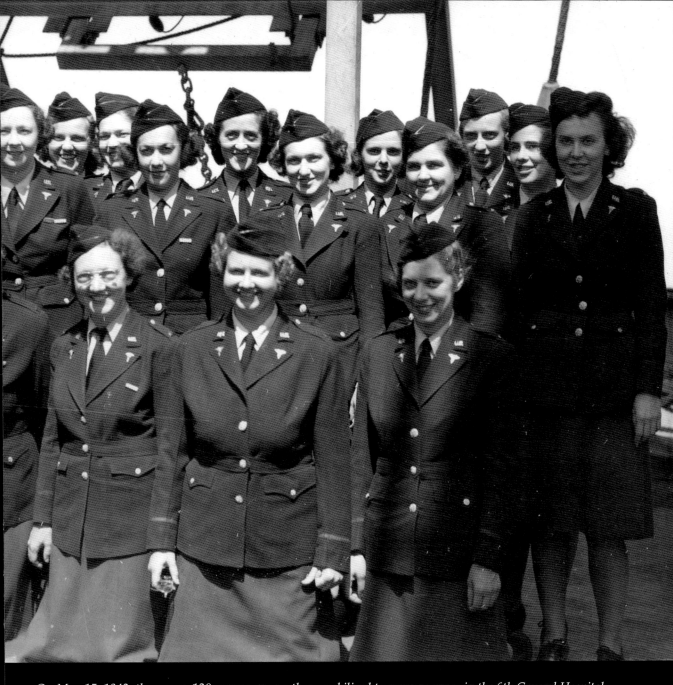

On May 15, 1942, there were 120 nurses among those mobilized to serve overseas in the 6th General Hospital; 71 were MGH School of Nursing graduates. Supervising the MASH OR units was (back row, sixth from the left) Helen J. "Coggie" Coghlan, RN, MSN, class of 1928. During the war, she is reported to have escorted General George S. Patton from the base hospital stating "General, you go run the Army. I'll run this hospital."

The Trustees of the hospital sent out a message to staff on December 31, 1942:

"Nurses have gone to war. The Armed Services will require a large percentage of all registered nurses. This means fewer for civilian needs. … The number of hospital floor nurses has also been greatly reduced by war. … It will be helpful if patients remember this and accept delays and deficiencies in service that in normal times would not be tolerated. This is one of the disciplines of wartime.

"With a depleted medical staff, fewer nurses, and a reduced number of employees in all departments, the Massachusetts General Hospital is trying to maintain its accustomed service to the general community."

Barrett, Katharine C. N-721173
6th General Hospital, APO 764,
U.S. Army.

Issued the following clothing:
3 pr. Anklets, wool
2 pr. Shoes, field
1 Jacket, field
1 Jacket, tropical worsted
1 Skirt, tropical worsted
4 Shirts, seersucker
4 Slacks, seersucker
4 pr. Panties, winter
4 pr. Stockings, wool
4 Vests, winter
4 Waists, wool
2 pr. Trousers, outer cover
1 pr. Trousers, wool liner
1 Jacket, pile
Turned in one blanket, wool, OD and issued one comforter.

Turned in one gas mask, diaphragm, and issued one light weight gas mask.

Placed on DS with the 81st Sta. Hosp. 14 January 1945, per par. 3, SO #9, Hq. 6th Gen. Hosp., dated 12 Jan. 1945.

Doris Knights
DORIS KNIGHTS
Major, Army Nurse Corps
Principal Chief Nurse

6th General Hospital APO 764 US Army

Relieved from DS with the 81st Sta. Hosp. and placed on DS with 50th Sta. Hosp., for an indefinite period, effective on or about 28 Feb. 1945, per par. 1, SO #28, Hq. 6th Gen. Hosp. dated 25 Feb. 1945.

Returned from DS to this station 6 May 1945.

Army of the United States of America

With the approval of the Secretary of War

Reserve Nurse   Katharine C. Barrett   N-721173 ,

of   120 High Street, Springfield, Mass. , *is hereby*

assigned to active service as Reserve Nurse, Army Nurse Corps, with the relative rank of

Second Lieutenant , *in conformity with Section 10, the National*

Defense Act as amended June 4, 1920 (41 Stat. 767), and will enter upon her duties on

March 2, 1942 , *after taking the oath prescribed by Section 1757 of the*

Revised Statutes of the United States. By authority of the Corps Area Commander:

W. T. MACMILLAN,
Colonel, A.G.D.,
Actg. Adjutant General.

For The Surgeon General.

Form 176
W. D., S. G. O.
(Revised Sept. 19, 1940)

GPO   16—18043

Unlike World War I, during which the nurses were listed as Red Cross Volunteers, the nurses of the 6th General Hospital in World War II received active duty orders into the Army Reserve Corps.

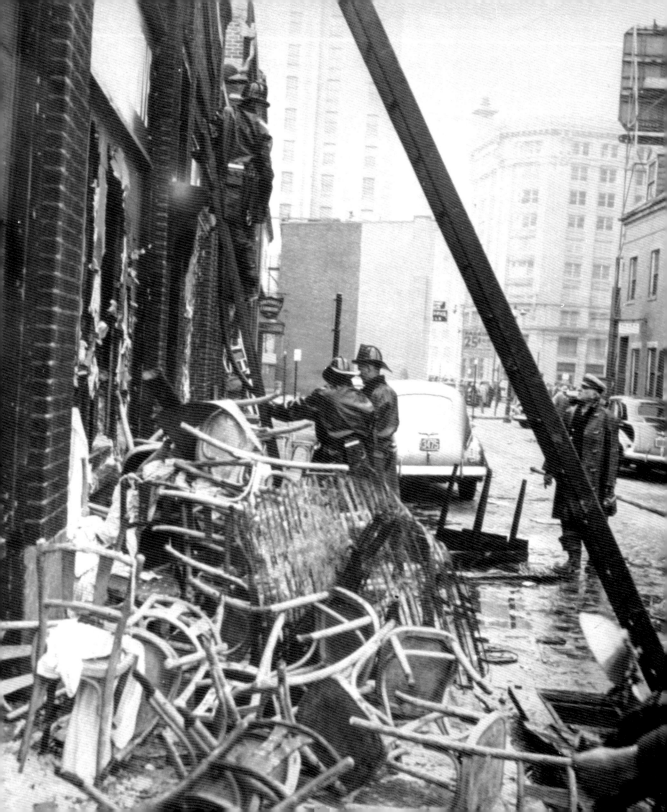

On November 28, 1942, nearly one thousand people crowded the Cocoanut Grove nightclub to party. Within an hour, a raging fire left 492 dead and hundreds injured and in Boston hospitals. MGH received 114 casualties: 39 living and 75 who were either dead on arrival or shortly after admission. The Cocoanut Grove fire demonstrated what being prepared really could mean in terms of saving lives. The hospital's response to those injured in the fire helped to create more effective resources for dealing with major emergencies in Boston. Fittingly, the hospital referred to its disaster plan internally as "Operation Cocoanut" for many years.

"I see that the papers estimate the damage at the Grove at $500,000, said the Assistant Superintendent of Nurses at the Massachusetts General Hospital [Ruth Sleeper], with a wry smile. The cost of those first three days in nursing, in doctors, in blood plasma and morphine, is almost beyond calculation. ...

One young girl in the Massachusetts General Hospital lost her father, mother, and fiancé. She didn't speak of her own feelings, but repeated over and over, I must get well; I must get out by Christmas. My little brother and sister will be alone for Christmas unless I get home."

— *The Atlantic Monthly*, March 1943

"The hospital had been 'Disaster Planning' in the event that the war reached American soil, so when the Cocoanut Grove fire occurred, we were ready to handle multiple casualties. That preparation alone may have saved who knows how many lives."

— Jean Ridgway Tienken, class of 1945,
who worked on the wards as a student
nurse the night of the Cocoanut Grove fire

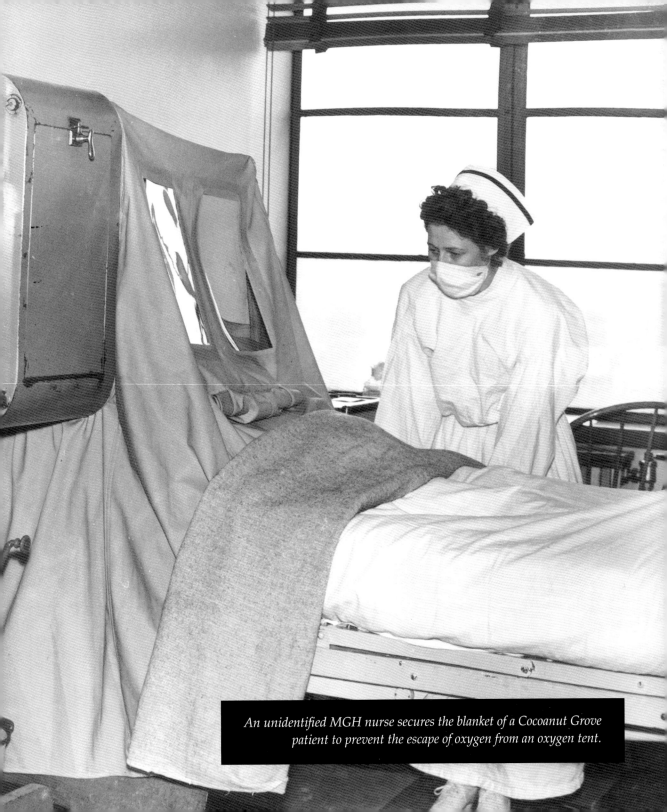

An unidentified MGH nurse secures the blanket of a Cocoanut Grove patient to prevent the escape of oxygen from an oxygen tent.

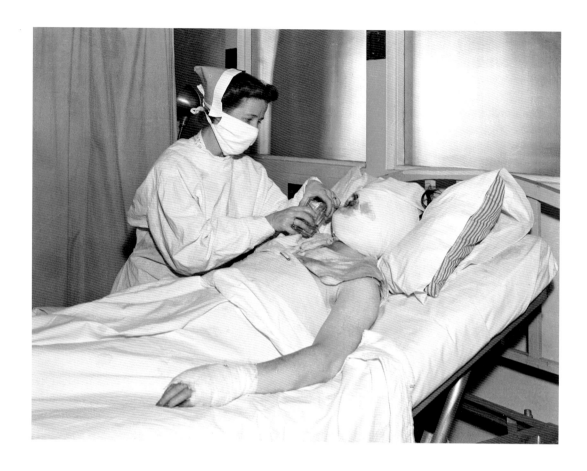

Post-World War II did not mean an increase in registered nurses to the hospital. Instead, there was an increase of auxiliary staff — nursing orderlies, licensed practical nurses and hospital aides. In order to make effective use of this staffing shift, to provide maximum care for the patients, improve the effectiveness of the head nurse, and promote harmonious relationships and job satisfaction for all staff, the Team Plan seemed to hold the answer. The basic concept centered around having every member of a care team think in terms of "our" patient versus "my" patient.

"Probably the chief bonus of the plan in nursing service situations was not so much the administrative advantages as it was the increased recognition of the value of every member of the team. "

— *Sylvia Perkins, RN, BS, MA, class of 1928, assistant director, MGH School of Nursing, 1941-1966, author of* A Centennial Review: The Massachusetts General Hospital School of Nursing

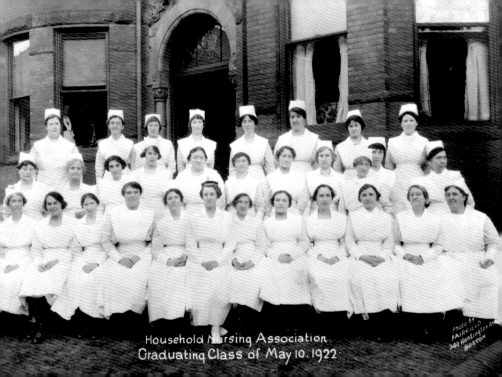

Household Nursing Association
Graduating Class of May 10, 1922

In 1951, MGH was the first Boston hospital to affiliate with the Household Nursing Association, which later became the Shepard-Gill School of Practical Nursing. In July 1970, the Shepard-Gill School was legally chartered as a part of the MGH, but remained wholly separate from the MGH School of Nursing. After it became part of the MGH, the curriculum became a model for other programs. As a 12-month program, it became a true career ladder program for those wanting to go into nursing. The vast majority of graduates of the Shepard-Gill School of Practical Nursing of the Massachusetts General Hospital continued their education toward an RN and advanced degrees in nursing. The 1982 opening of the MGH Institute of Health Professions Graduate Program in Nursing created a philosophical problem of educating nurses at both an LPN and a master's level. In 1984, the practical nursing program was closed after training 4,464 graduates.

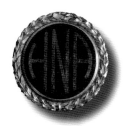

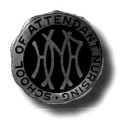

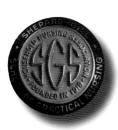

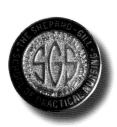

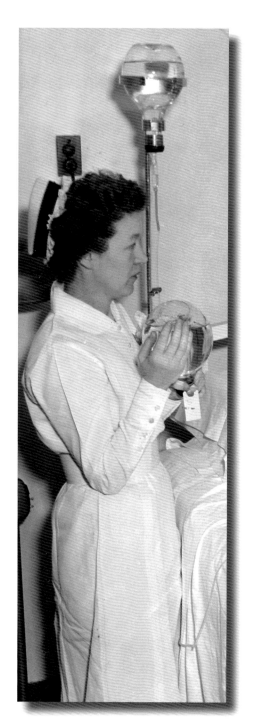

In 1953, nursing shifted to the much shorter 40-hour work week: "The standard work week for graduate and licensed practical nurses will be reduced to forty hours. There will be no reduction in salary for those who change from forty-four to forty hours… Permanent evening and night staff nurses will continue to work a forty-hour week and will receive a proportionate increase in salary … the time worked beyond forty hours by those on the weekly payroll will be regarded as overtime."

— *From a July 2, 1953, Ruth Sleeper memo to graduate and licensed practical nurses*

Miriam (Mim) Huggard, RN, class of 1931, supervisor of the Phillips House Nursing Service

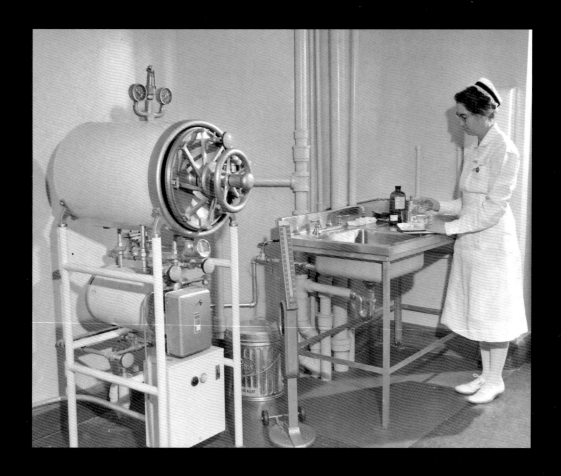

The autoclave, although time consuming, was the most efficient way to sterilize equipment on the units. With the advent of individualized packages of sterile syringes and needles, the time saved to provide nursing care to the patients was invaluable.

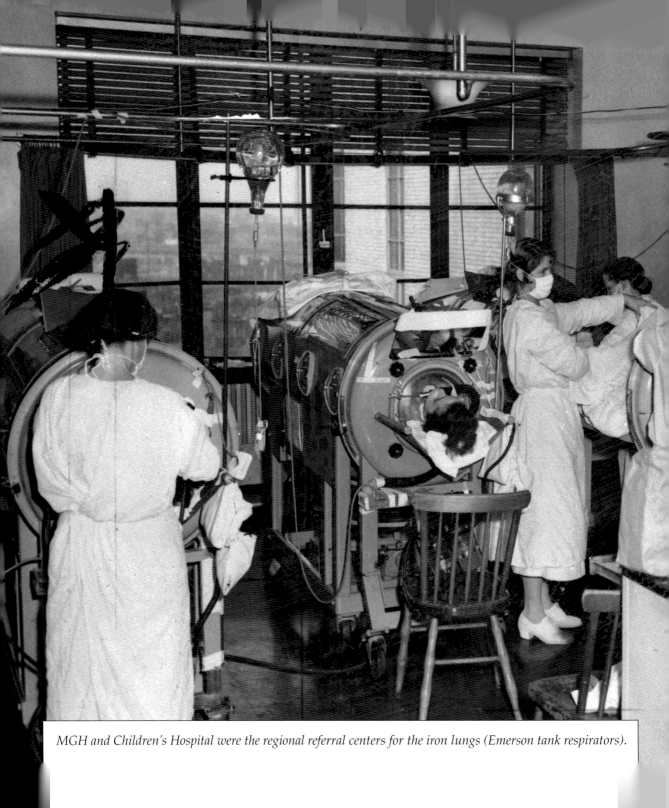

MGH and Children's Hospital were the regional referral centers for the iron lungs (Emerson tank respirators).

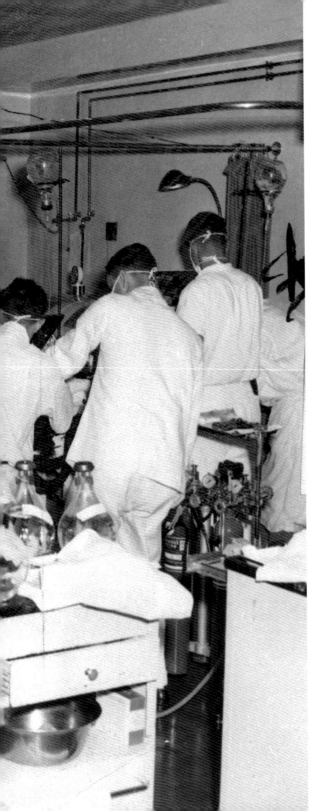

In 1955, before the Salk vaccine became available, an epidemic of poliomyelitis occurred in the Boston area, taxing the facilities of the MGH and its Nursing Service. The ninth floor of the White Building was quickly emptied to set up a respirator unit, and "Polio Teams" were organized to provide round-the-clock care. In total, 428 patients were admitted with polio in some form — 376 adults and 52 children. Of those, 73 adults and eight children were in respirators for varying periods of time. As of January 1956, there were still 30 patients in respirators. Patricia Beckles, RN, a pediatric staff nurse, recalls, "If they could breathe for a few minutes on their own you could take them out of the respirator for short periods. I can remember the look of joy on their faces while they were out, and the look of anxiety when they had to return to the respirator."

The novel approach to the polio epidemic led to the development of Respiratory Care and also the concept of the Intensive Care Unit (ICU). After White (Building) 9 was closed as a polio ward in 1957 or 1958, respirator patients were cared for in single rooms on the Surgical Service floors [mostly White 6 and 7] and on the Neurosurgical Service floor [White 11]. Medical Service patients were primarily housed on Bulfinch 3. Private patients — those who had their own doctors and were not cared for by the house staff — were cared for in single rooms in the Baker Building and the Phillips House. In 1961, the hospital opened a five-bed Respiratory Unit — later renamed the Respiratory Intensive Care Unit (RICU) — in Phillips House. In 1969 the RICU moved to a 10-bed unit in the Jackson/Gray Building.

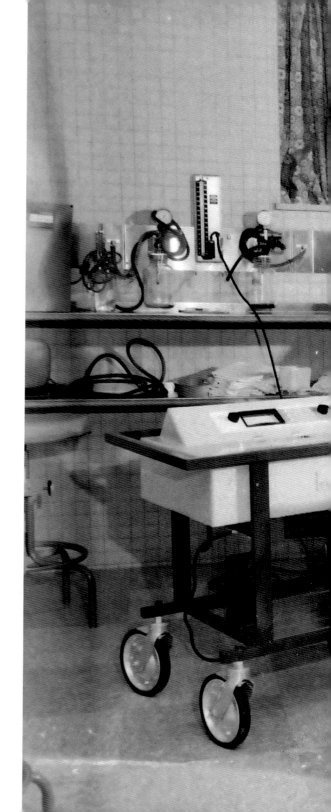

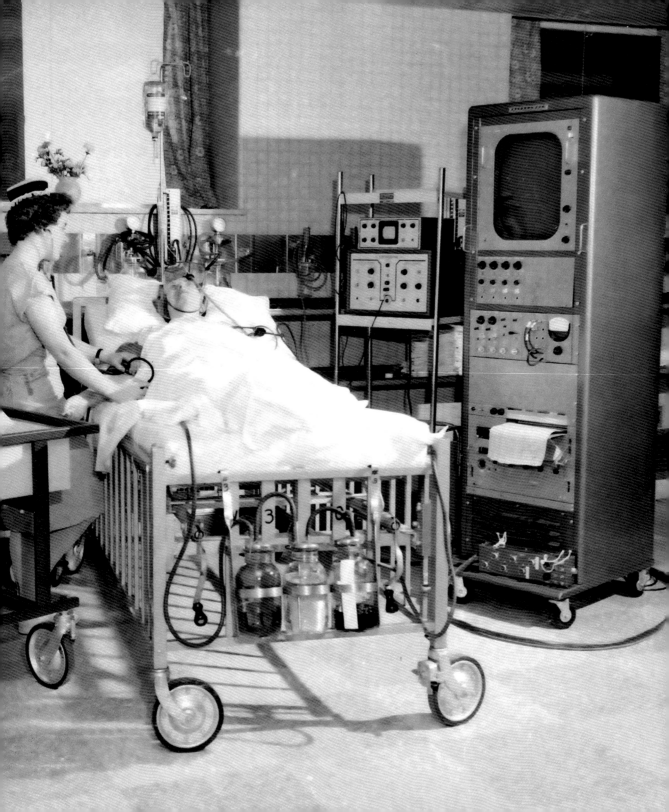

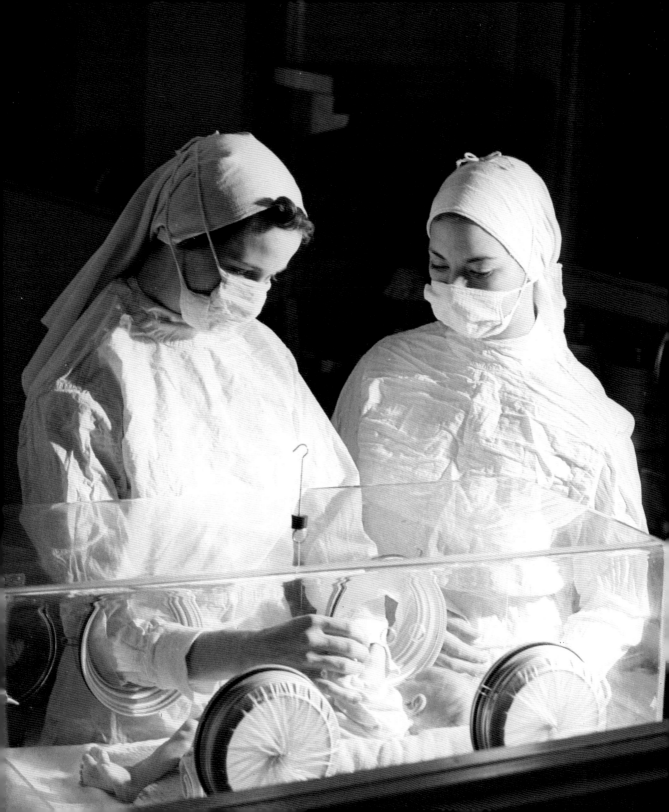

"As the acuity of our patients grew, in order to better serve our patients added technology was imperative. New techniques and equipment were developed, enabling us to provide the very best care available. I witnessed and participated in the transformation of the newborn nursery into the Neonatal Intensive Care Unit, among the earliest units of its kind."

— Patricia Beckles, RN, Pediatric staff nurse

Prompted by a devastating plane crash in 1961, two years later, MGH became the first general hospital in the United States to establish and operate a medical station at an international airport. The Logan Airport Medical Station offered health services to residents of East Boston, airport employees and several million travelers annually.

Five full-time nurses provided 24-hour coverage, and in 1968 they established direct communication with the MGH through a telecommunication system that made advice and necessary physician orders immediately available. This is believed to have been the first use of telemedicine for general patient care and physical diagnosis.

The medical station was connected by two-way television with the MGH Emergency Ward. Patients were triaged and treated by a staff of nurse practitioners, with medical consultation available through a television circuit.

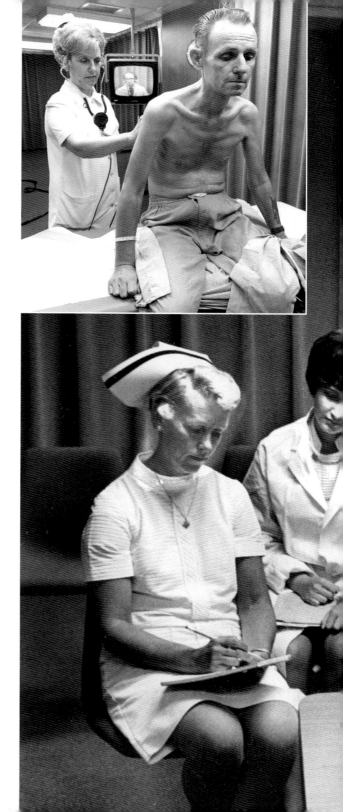

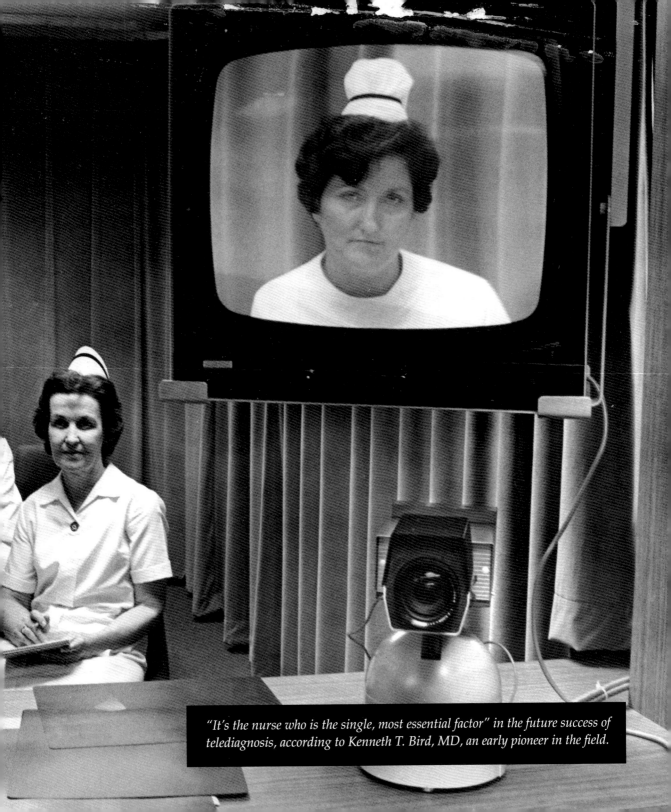

"It's the nurse who is the single, most essential factor" in the future success of *telediagnosis, according to Kenneth T. Bird, MD, an early pioneer in the field.*

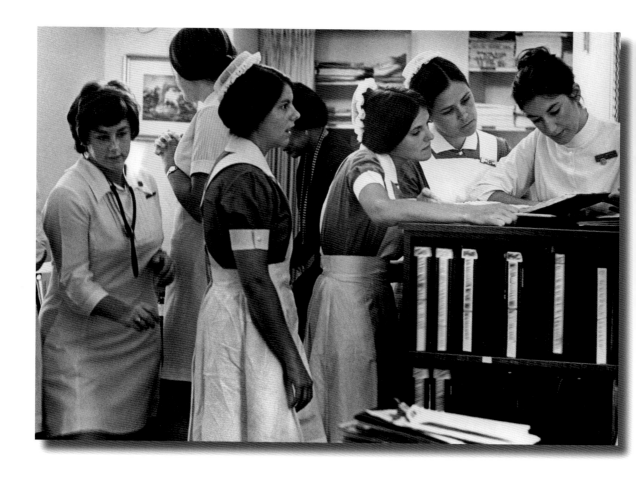

The 1960s brought great change to the Nursing Service, due largely to the rapid growth of intensive and special care units and the 1965 introduction of Medicare. Once Medicare became fully implemented, nurses (versus students) were then required to deliver care. This impacted the clinical assignment of the hospital's nursing students and resulted in a dramatic increase in the number of staff nurses needed to deliver care. In 1960, MGH had 958 licensed inpatient beds and 278 registered staff nurses. By 1970, the number of beds had increased by only 127 to 1,085, but there were 650 registered staff nurses.

Also in 1965, a major shift in nursing education occurred. In an effort to provide direction for improving both the system of nursing education and the service of nursing practitioners, the American Nurses Association (ANA) issued a statement on the educational preparation required for nursing. In doing so, the organization affirmed its belief that unless all nursing education was upgraded, nurses would be handicapped in providing advanced patient care made possible by expanding scientific knowledge. In essence, the ANA took the position that the education of those who work in nursing should take place in institutions of learning within the general system of education, and that the minimal preparation for beginning professional nursing practice should

be a baccalaureate degree. Diploma versus degreed education remained a topic of national debate for the nursing profession throughout the 1960s. The MGH Trustees and administrators shared a concern about the future of the hospital's own nurse training program and began weighing options that would offer control over education quality.

The Ether Dome and other amphitheaters throughout the hospital were used as classrooms for student nurses.

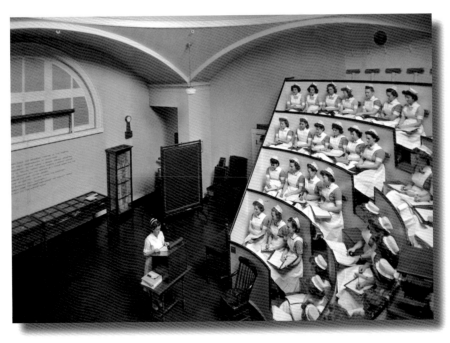

The 1960s also marked a time when the United States had become very involved in the war in Vietnam. In the wake of World War II, the United States passed the National Defense Act of 1947, in which nursing was declared an essential service. Given the subsequent expansion of the military nursing service and increased nursing participation in the civil defense program, MGH hosted a pilot program specifically to train nurses for Vietnam.

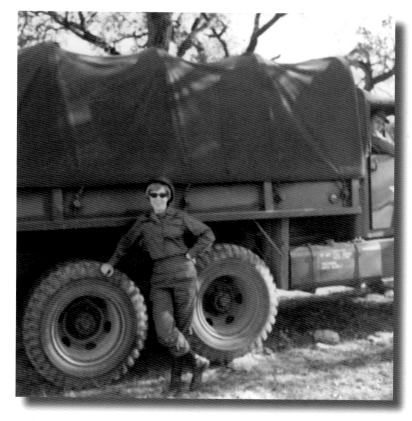

Roberta Keene Nemeskal, class of 1969, is pictured during field training at Fort Sam Houston in Texas, just months after graduation. As commissioned officers in the U.S. Army, nurses were considered "soldiers first, nurses second." Their six-week officer training consisted of didactic classroom lecture and field training, which included convoy transport, MASH/Medical Unit assembly, combat trauma triage, M-16 shooting precision, gas-mask training, and literally living in Army tents.

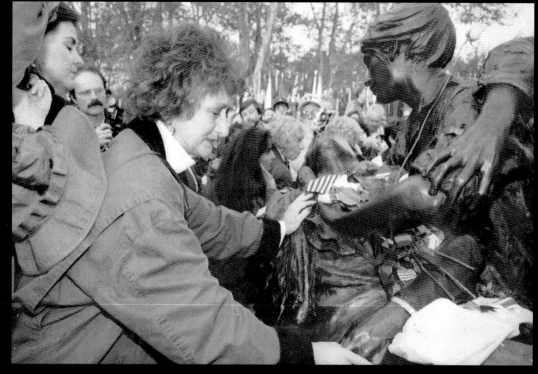

Barbara Teixeira Goral, class of 1967, at the dedication of the Vietnam Women's Memorial, located on the National Mall in Washington, D.C. Approximately 10,000 women — most nurses, including Goral — served in Vietnam. As she stated in the Boston Herald, *"Even though our numbers were small, our sacrifices were tremendous." Photo courtesy of the* Boston Herald.

"As the Vietnam War escalated, the U.S. Army enhanced nursing recruitment efforts through its U.S. Army Student Nurse Program. Nursing students entering their last one or two years of nursing school were recruited as inactive enlisted personnel receiving Private grade [E-2] monthly pay. Following their nursing school graduation, participants were commissioned as officers in the Army Nurse Corps and served on active duty for two to three years."

"I was the first unit teacher in Pediatrics and had five diversified units, so there was no well-traveled path before me. It was a challenge to try to develop the newly created role designed for an individual who would have a lesser scope of responsibility."

— Carolyn Wortman, RN,
unit teacher at MGH

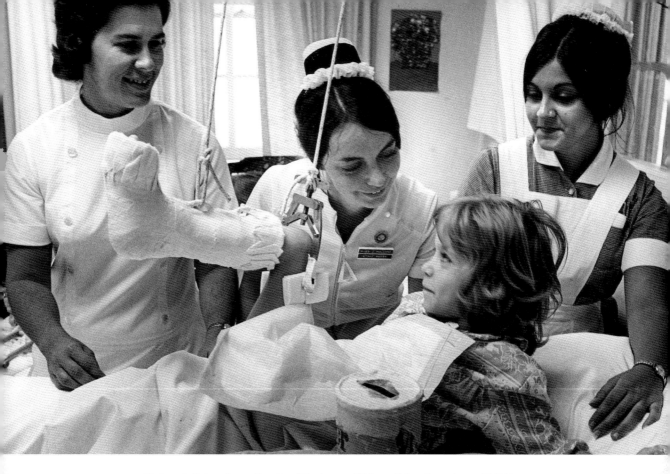

Pictured (l. to r.) are Carolyn Wortman, RN, unit teacher, class of 1954; Janice Mulcahy, RN, staff nurse, class of 1972; and an unidentified student.

In the late 1960s, MGH introduced the concept of having unit teachers available on the patient care units, an approach that was later duplicated throughout the country. The basic premise was that nurses had to change, think, process, advocate and constantly learn. A centralized staff education department could not foster this development for each individual. The unit teacher was responsible to the clinical leader on the unit, who supervised new graduates. This had a positive impact on staff retention, which had become a major issue.

"I told Dr. Knowles [MGH general director] that I would only take the job if it was as chief of Nursing Service so that nursing would be on the same level as the other services that had chiefs. One of my first acts as chief was to change the name to the Department of Nursing, to better reflect the patient care, teaching, and research aspects of the profession."

— *Mary Macdonald, RN, MA, FAAN*
from an interview conducted in 1997

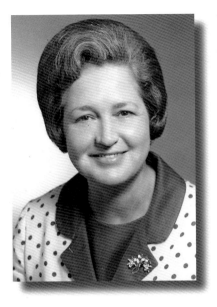

Mary Macdonald, RN, MA, FAAN,

was an author, researcher, activist and nursing leader who earned a reputation as a visionary throughout her four-decade career. A 1942 graduate of the MGH School of Nursing, Macdonald began her career in academia, and later returned to the MGH as director of Analytic Studies in Nursing. In 1968 she became chief of the Nursing Service, a position she held until 1983. It was a time of social and value-laden revolutions in the United States, with the start of the Vietnam War and the civil rights movement. Within the hospital, the number of intensive care units was increasing dramatically, having a profound impact on the recruitment and responsibilities of nurses. She described the profession of nursing at that time as being in a "becoming stage," and her goal was to establish a system of delivering care that would permit the nurse to nurse, in the true sense of the professional mission. "Our objectives will be to … create an environment in which the nurse can function as a participating member of the total health team." Macdonald was also responsible for broadening the scope of nurses by introducing the unit teacher role, a move that was replicated in hospitals across the country. By her own assessment, though, "My greatest accomplishment was the freedom I gave to staff with the idea that no matter where you were in the line you had something to offer."

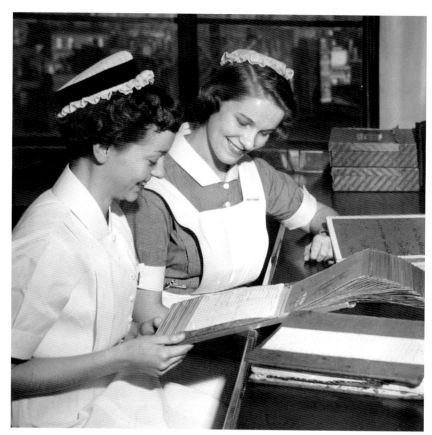

The Kardex was a frame that included a form for each patient with space for all of the information a nurse needed for care delivery. It was the only place that the nurse could write a note each shift.

Early in Macdonald's tenure, there was a day-long colloquium with about 250 nurses in attendance, 200 of them from the MGH. This was a day to share ideas and find innovative ways in which the nurse could improve patient care and identify their role in the health delivery system. From this colloquium came STAT, which stands for "Start Taking Action Today." One of the innovations by STAT was the addition of nursing notes to the medical chart. Prior to this, the nursing notes were in the Kardex only and the medical record was for the physician notes. The nurses who were part of STAT wanted to humanize the hospitals and expand the nursing focus on the patient.

"Ms. Macdonald made the change that was perhaps waiting to happen. Not merely a pass-through but a change, a good call to action, to care, to think, to improvise, to triage, to do what was right for the patient at that moment, not what had been tradition. She felt that change was not to be feared. Orientations and education were where nurses could learn and be mentored and that included leadership mentoring for head nurses. So that by the end of her tenure as the hospital moved to specialized units, the head nurse had a true leadership position. And staff on the units became experts to give the best possible care to the patient."

— *Ruth Dempsey, RN,*
retired nurse manager,
Thoracic Surgical Unit

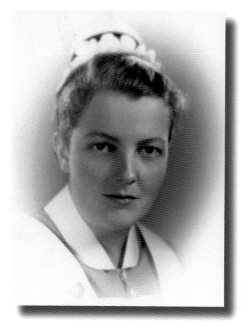

Ruth Farrisey, RN

In 1968, MGH introduced a pediatric nurse practitioner program, only the second in the country.

"Around 1960, Dr. John Stoeckle asked if a nurse clinic could be run in his medical clinic on Friday afternoons. It expanded to Wednesday and Friday afternoons and reinforced nurses to be the pivotal person for the patient and the family.

"Then in late 1964, Dr. Jack Connolly, a pediatrician, asked for a meeting to discuss the development of the pediatric nurse practitioner program after a model of the one he visited in Colorado. It started with a pediatric practitioner in 1968, as the pediatric physicians were the first to want the nurse in an expanded role.

"In 1970, the adult nurse practitioner program started. [We] had to separate pediatric from adult as the emphasis of the adult was on chronic disease follow up, and in pediatrics it was on wellness and maintenance of wellness before looking at illness. By the mid-'70s, the Primary Care Physician program combined with the Adult Nurse Practitioner program. Protocols were written by the nurses to reinforce the role of the Nurse Practitioner. The doctors clearly were interested and supportive so there was never a protocol rejected by the Executive Committee."

— *Ruth Farrisey, RN, class of 1938, associate director,*
Department of Nursing for Ambulatory Care, October 2002

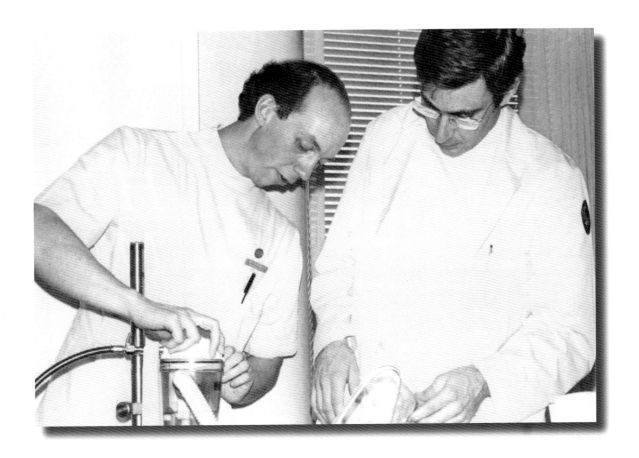

The McLean Hospital Training School for Nurses graduated its first class in 1886, and throughout the years saw an ever-increasing number of male students. If you were male and wanted to be a nurse, you went to McLean, at that time the only school in the area that accepted male students. The students had clinical rotations at MGH along with the MGH School of Nursing students. The MGH School of Nursing did not enroll men until 1969, after the McLean program had closed. The class that entered in 1969 included three men, and by the class of 1977, eight percent of the class was male.

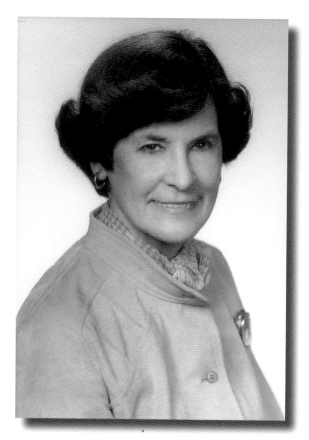

Ada Plumer, RN, class of 1938

Intravenous therapy (IV) provides an enduring example of a rapidly-growing MGH service provided by nurses that also left its mark nationally and internationally. The service started in 1940 at the MGH with one nurse, Ada Plumer, RN, class of 1938. In her first year, she answered 300 calls for IV therapy. By 1961, the service had grown to a staff of nine nurses who carried out some 42,000 procedures for patients in the Phillips House and the Baker Memorial Building. Believed to have been the first person ever to hold the title "IV nurse," in 1973 Plumer cofounded the National Intravenous Therapy Association, now the Infusion Nurses Society.

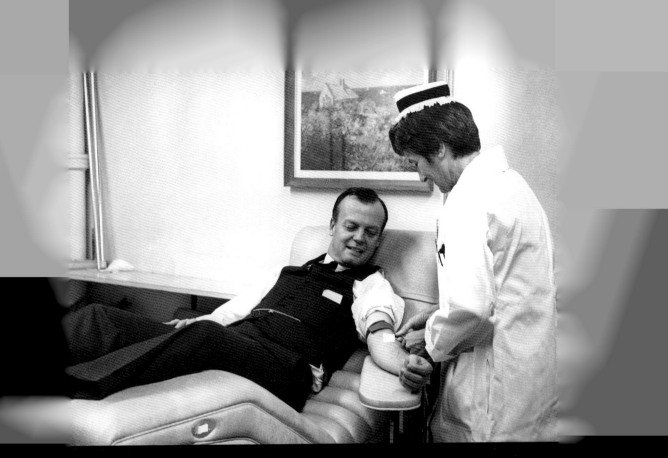

John Knowles, MD, former MGH general director, donating blood

"In the late '60s and early '70s, Plumer recognized the need for IV therapy information beyond MGH. Teams were starting to form and were floundering for information. She and Marge Knight, supervisor of IV Therapy at Johns Hopkins, had communicated and decided to start a national organization so that quality standards for the practice could be established."

As early as 1917, nursing education at the MGH had already created a coordinated program with Simmons College. This was the first college connection started by a training school in New England. The MGH catalogues each year offered entering students the option of this program. The program continued until 1934.

However, the desire to link the MGH with a collegiate program remained. In 1943, Ruth Sleeper reactivated the search for an affiliation by approaching not only Harvard and Radcliffe but also MIT, Wellesley, Simmons, Northeastern, Boston University and the Massachusetts State College in Amherst. The challenge in creating a coordinated program was that the MGH school was not ready or willing to give up full control of the school to any academic institution.

From this work affiliations were started. The first in 1945 was the Coordinated Program with Radcliffe College, which survived, with major changes in 1959, until it closed in 1966.

Hood College in Maryland sought affiliation in the same way, and that program started at the MGH in 1948 and closed in 1962. Both of these programs had separate faculty at the MGH, so in 1950 Simmons College resumed having the MGH School of Nursing for all nursing-related clinical and classroom work. This program graduated its final class in 1959.

The final effort to join forces with a collegiate program came in 1962 with the creation of the "Alternate Program" with Northeastern University. This was a three-year program leading to a diploma from the MGH and an associate degree from Northeastern. Students spent the majority of the freshman year as full-time students at Northeastern and in the late spring arrived at the MGH as full-time students for the remainder of the program. They attended one evening course at Northeastern each quarter to satisfy the degree requirements.

The program had a separate faculty at MGH but shared clinical rotations with the other MGH School of Nursing students. The only way to know there was a different program was that the Alternate Program students wore a red and black ribbon above their name tag. Only two classes entered this program, which closed in 1966 after Northeastern opened its own nursing program.

The MGH School of Nursing had not been willing to give up control or the MGH name, and it was felt that no hospital could control a collegiate program in nursing. Miss Sleeper never gave up and told students in the Alternate Program as they were finishing that, "someday the MGH will be degree-granting." She was a strong advocate and set the tone for the MGH seeking degree-granting status and the early foundation for the MGH Institute of Health Professions.

"As the first unit teacher in the Respiratory ICU, I was privileged to be a mentor, supervisor and educator to the new nurses in the unit. Their transition to competent respiratory ICU nurses was facilitated at a rate much faster than before and with much less stress!"

— *Barbara Teixeira Goral, RN,*
class of 1967, unit teacher

In 1986, master's-prepared cardiovascular-pulmonary, oncology and gerontology clinical nurse specialists (CNSs) were introduced at MGH. The CNSs complemented and collaborated with unit teachers, orientating newly hired nurses as well as planning and conducting in-service education and continuing education for nurses throughout the Department of Nursing. Initially, the CNSs were service-based, following a caseload of patients and families dealing with specialty-related physiological and psychosocial problems. The CNSs also collaborated with nursing leadership and other disciplines to conduct quality assurance programs, infuse research findings into practice (the precursor to today's evidence-based practice movement) and create innovative clinical programs. After a centralized "Performance-Based Development Program (PBDP)" and then a model of staff nurse preceptor orientation was adopted for nursing orientation, the unit teachers became "clinical teachers" and ultimately "clinical educators," who were centralized in the new Center for Clinical and Professional Development (1996). In a parallel transition, CNSs became unit-based in order to maximize the local infusion of expert clinical, teaching, and research knowledge and skills.

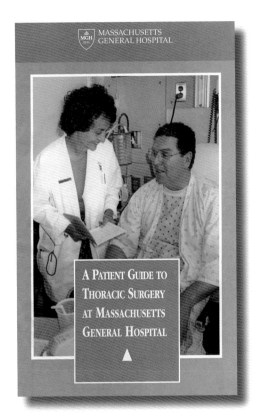

Pictured above, Stephanie Macaluso, RN, BSN, MSN, MGH Institute of Health Professions class of 1988, was a unit teacher and later a clinical nurse specialist in Thoracic Surgery. In 1996, she became the first recipient of the MGH Award for Expertise in Clinical Practice, renamed the Stephanie M. Macaluso, RN, Excellence in Clinical Practice Award after she lost her battle with cancer.

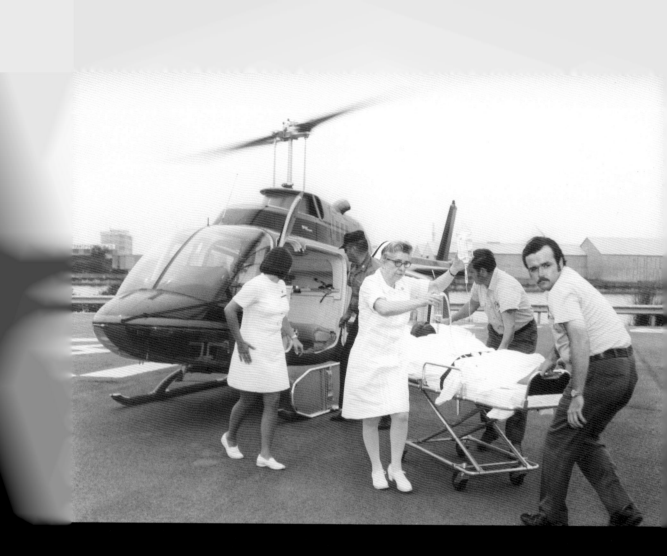

The need to transport patients safely from other hospitals for specialized care
required a team effort, with the nurse as a key player. During the 1970s, the
RICU specialized in the care of patients with acute respiratory failure (ARF)
and/or adult respiratory distress syndrome (ARDS), and had one of the few
hospital-based ECMO (extracorporeal membrane oxygenation) centers in
the United States. Safe transport of these critically ill patients from outside
hospitals to the MGH was at best difficult and often unsafe.

"Appreciating these obstacles, Dr. Michael Rie, one of the attending physicians in the Respiratory ICU, organized a critical care transport service," said Roberta Keene Nemeskal, RN, class of 1969. "Ambulance services were contracted with a privately owned ambulance company that happened to have an Advanced Life Care Support in its ambulance fleet [rare in the 1970s], as the common Basic Life Support ambulance would not have accommodated the needed equipment for mechanical ventilation, resuscitation and critical care staff required for safe patient transport."

"The Neonatal Transport Team was first started in 1972," recalls Pat Beckles, RN. "The original team consisted of a nurse and a doctor. In the middle of the night, when we got a call, we would grab a bag with a few syringes and medicines and off we would go in an ambulance not knowing what to expect. We taped the stethoscope to the baby's chest, as they had no monitors back then."

Nearly 40 years later, "the team today is comprised of a registered nurse, a registered therapist and a physician," says Anita Carew, RN. "They comprise a traveling intensive care unit equipped for any emergency. It's not uncommon for extremely premature babies (weighing less than one pound) to be transported to MGH for care. We take great pride in the safe, expert care we provide during every transport."

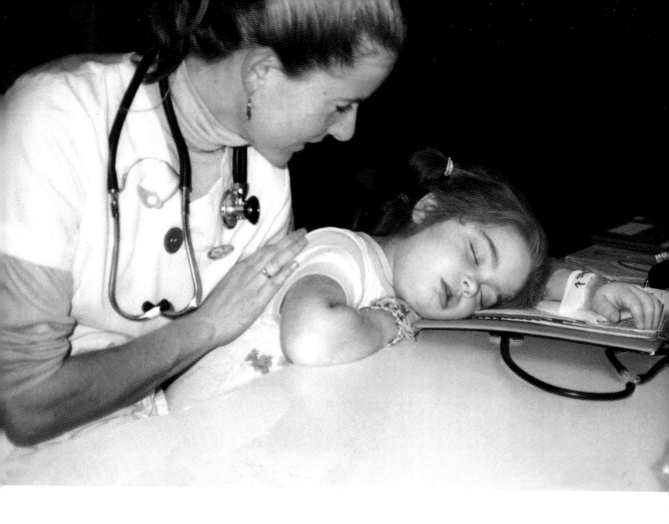

By the 1970s, primary nursing was the practice for the MGH Pediatric Service. As a patient and family arrived on the unit, a nurse would take responsibility for the family as a primary nurse with others as secondary nurses. This allowed the family and the child to bond with "their nurse," who could give the best possible care and be available for the child and family during the admission and any future admissions to the unit. In other areas of nursing the concept was just starting to be considered.

"When primary nursing came into being in the 1970s, it reflected all the thoughts and ideas I had from this period. I came into pediatrics to care not just for the child but the family. As a nurse it is rewarding when you see the child recover, saddening when a child is lost and enlightening because you always learn from the experience."

— Marlene Norton, RN,
class of 1961

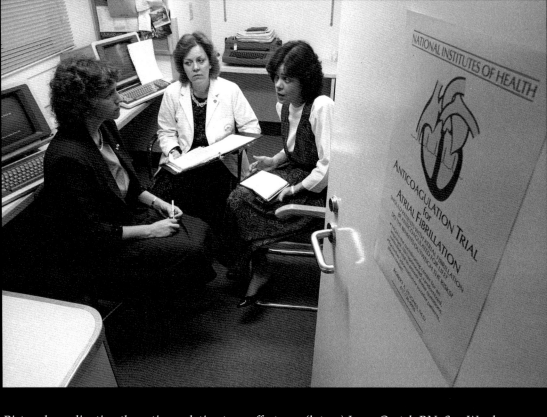

Pictured coordinating the anticoagulation team efforts are (l. to r.) Lynn Oertel, RN; Sue Ward Maraventano, RN; and Mary Sheehan, RN, as they reviewed patient results and strategized for the coming week. The three and the service's first nurse, Mary Welch-Costantino, RN, were still working at MGH into 2011. Photograph is by Jeff Thiebauth.

Another example of a successful nurse-driven approach to care can be found in the MGH Anticoagulation Management Service (AMS), among the largest and oldest anticoagulation clinics in the world. Established in 1969 in a cardiology practice, the Anticoagulant Therapy Unit (ATU) traditionally focused on the outpatient management of warfarin therapy. In 1972, the ATU became fully computerized, including implementation of a dose algorithm for clinical decision support. In 1982, the ATU hired its first registered nurse, Maureen Welch-Costantino, RN, to assist the existing secretary with patient management. Today, the AMS has a team of 14 nurses and four administrative support personnel.

During the 1990s, the AMS provided rich opportunities for investigation and study. Collectively, this research significantly added to the body of evidence around anticoagulation safety and quality, including insights for improved management. Studies helped create new standards of care to prevent stroke in atrial fibrillation patients, explored therapeutic safety boundaries, assessed patient quality of life issues and more.

Circa 2005, AMS experienced significant growth and development with a strategic move into the Department of Nursing, creating key leadership positions, evolving staff roles and responsibilities, and expanding clinical services. This move not only facilitated a seamless transition of care from hospital to home but continues to help validate and improve warfarin management. Significant changes in the infrastructure to support this work, including the implementation of a primary nurse model of care and a new information system, contribute to greater emphasis on patient and family-focused care, along with achieving improved outcomes.

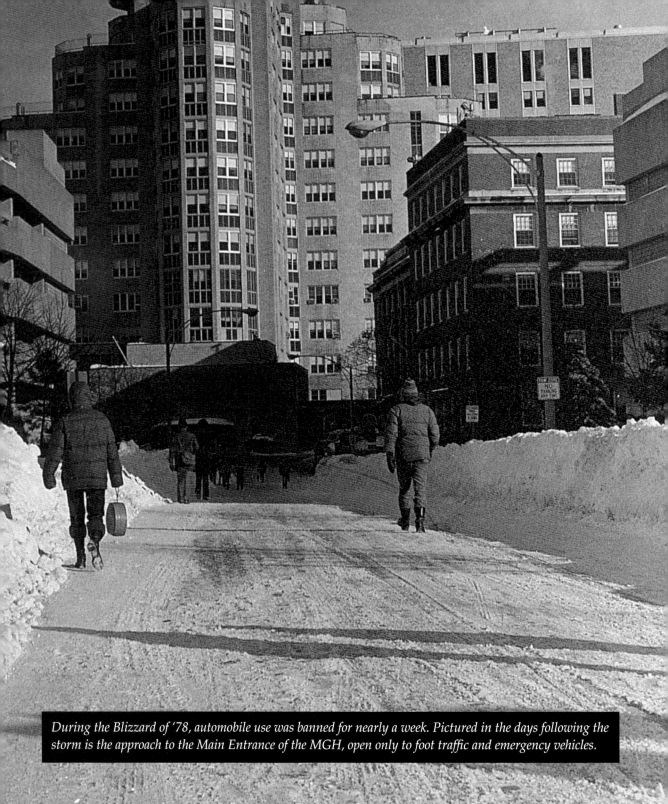

During the Blizzard of '78, automobile use was banned for nearly a week. Pictured in the days following the storm is the approach to the Main Entrance of the MGH, open only to foot traffic and emergency vehicles.

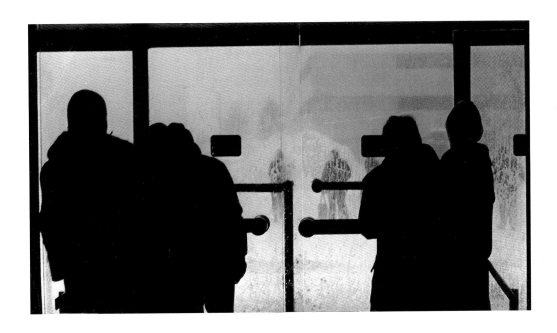

The Blizzard of '78 was one of the biggest snowstorms ever to hit Boston. With some 30 inches of snow, wind gusts exceeding 60 miles per hour and snowdrifts 15 feet high, the city was brought to a complete standstill. "During the blizzard some of the nurses were stranded at the hospital for five days. The National Guard was instrumental in bringing some nurses to work. When both the power and auxiliary power went down, there were seven children on respirators who had to be hand ventilated for several hours. They all survived due to the incredible diligence of the staff. We had no hot meals, and the parents went to the kitchen and made and served sandwiches to both the staff and patients. The camaraderie of everyone turned this crisis into a workable and safe situation for both nurses and patients."

— Anne Sheetz, RN,
former chair, Pediatric Nursing

In 1981, the MGH made the difficult decision to close its School of Nursing. This was an event years in the making. As the School celebrated its centennial in 1973, its future seemed uncertain, as nursing education was rapidly shifting to a collegiate model. Ruth Sleeper, RN, class of 1922, former director of the School of Nursing and Department of Nursing, urged John Knowles, MD, the hospital's general director, to have the MGH petition the Massachusetts Board of Higher Education to confer degree-granting authority to the Massachusetts General Hospital Educational Division.

In 1977, the Board granted MGH's request, paving the way for postgraduate certificate and master's-degree-level programs to be offered by the MGH. Natalie Petzold, RN, the director of the School of Nursing, cochaired a committee to explore degree-granting status and the feasibility of establishing a freestanding interdisciplinary graduate school. She said, "It was sometimes hard to go to a meeting and think long term, because it really would bring an end to the School of Nursing as we knew it."

In fact, this was exactly true. In 1980, the hospital formally established the interdisciplinary MGH Institute of Health Professions, and a year later the celebrated Massachusetts General Hospital School of Nursing graduated its last class and closed its doors.

A new MGH era in nursing education began in 1982, when the Institute's Graduate Program in Nursing admitted its first entry-level master's students. This was the country's first hospital-based graduate degree program and one of the first to enroll baccalaureate-prepared individuals with no prior experience or education in nursing.

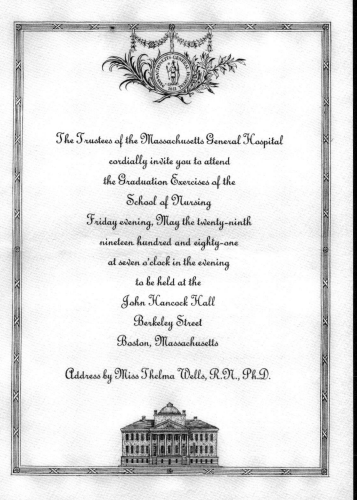

The Trustees of the Massachusetts General Hospital
cordially invite you to attend
the Graduation Exercises of the
School of Nursing
Friday evening, May the twenty-ninth
nineteen hundred and eighty-one
at seven o'clock in the evening
to be held at the
John Hancock Hall
Berkeley Street
Boston, Massachusetts

Address by Miss Thelma Wells, R.N., Ph.D.

"It's almost as if all generations of graduates are with us on this night ... the ghosts of classes past."

— Thelma Wells, RN, PhD, FAAN class of 1962, speaker at th[e] final MGH School of Nursing Graduation Ceremony, June 198[1]

From 1873 to the last graduating class in 1981, the MGH School of Nursing graduated 7,032 nurses.

I graduated from the School of Nursing in 1963 and the Nurse Practitioner Program in the '70s but I never worked harder than I did at the MGH Institute for my Master of Science in Nursing."

— *Jo Birdsey, RN, MSN, class of 1963*

The first nursing students graduated from the MGH Institute of Health Professions Graduate Program in Nursing in 1985 as clinical nurse specialists. Since then, the MGH Institute has changed its focus to educating nurse practitioners and creating pathways for existing nurses to earn advanced degrees. In 2008, the Institute received program approval for both an accelerated Bachelor of Science in Nursing and a Doctor of Nursing Practice.

In 2009, the MGH Institute's Graduate Program in Nursing was officially renamed the MGH Institute School of Nursing. Graduates of the Institute continue the tradition of the generations that came before them, making their mark on the nursing profession locally, nationally and internationally.

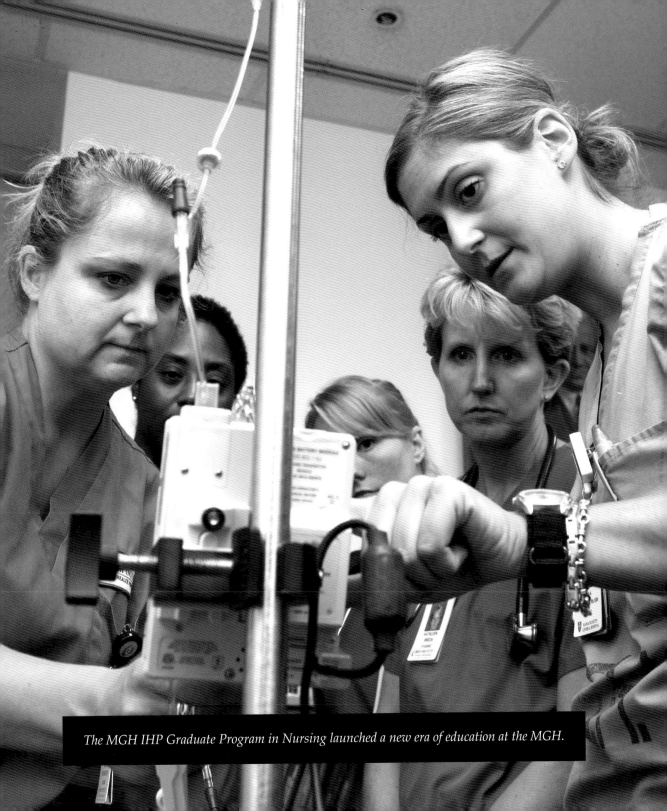

The MGH IHP Graduate Program in Nursing launched a new era of education at the MGH.

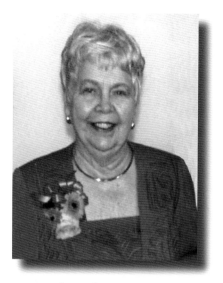

Yvonne L. Munn, RN, MSN, a native of Edmonton, Canada, had a nursing career that spanned more than 40 years. Her first nursing leadership position was as a science instructor at Edmonton General School of Nursing, and two years later she assumed the assistant director of nursing position at Alberta's Medicine Hat General Hospital and education director for that hospital's school of nursing. In 1956, she moved to the United States when she accepted a position as assistant director of nursing services at Sharp Memorial Hospital in San Diego, Calif. Munn continued her leadership journey at Presbyterian-St. Luke's Hospital in Chicago, Ill. She began as the Division of Nursing's assistant chairperson for education and research in 1969. By the time she left, eight years later, she held the positions of assistant vice president for nursing at Rush Presbyterian–St. Luke's Medical Center and associate dean of Rush College of Nursing. Prior to her position as associate general director and director of nursing at MGH, she was vice president for nursing services, vice president for patient services and vice president for patient systems and evaluation at Methodist Hospitals of Dallas in Texas.

Upon her retirement, she acknowledged her respect for the commitment of MGH nurses saying, "[They] will do what they have always done through many transitions — hold to their ideals and initiate and support the changes that must be made." In 1993, the Department of Nursing established the annual Yvonne L. Munn Lecture, and in 1997, the Yvonne L. Munn Nursing Research awards in her honor.

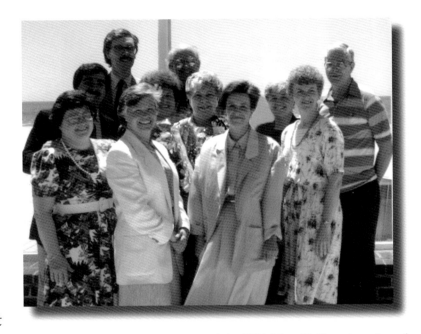

Yvonne L. Munn, RN, was presented the 1991 Mary B. Conceison Award at the Annual Meeting of the Massachusetts Organization of Nurse Executives (MONE). Prior to her death in 1981, Conceison was director of Professional Relations at the Massachusetts Hospital Association. Over the course of her career, her contributions to the profession of nursing in Massachusetts were numerous and highly regarded. The award in her name recognizes nurse leaders who follow in her footsteps. Pictured at the annual meeting are members of the Nursing Executive Team (l. to r.) front row: Christina Graf, RN; Mary Connaughton, RN; Jeanette Ives Erickson, RN; Sally Millar, RN; second row: Gary Schweon, RN; Deanna Perlmutter, RN; Yvonne Munn, RN; Joan Fitzmaurice, RN; third row: Tom Smith, RN; Ed Coakley, RN; and Munn's husband Roger.

In the 1960s, minorities in the United States were fighting for their civil rights. At MGH there were few nurses of color on the professional nursing staff and even fewer in positions of authority. In 1991, a nurse recruiter named Beverly Cummings decided to find out why, and tried to find a way to increase their numbers. With her encouragement, a group of black staff nurses formed the MGH Minority Nurse Task Force. Members met with nurse managers to discuss strategies and tactics that would have a positive impact on the larger organizational commitment to diversity, specifically related to hiring goals. The committee set out not only to recruit new minority nurses, but to increase opportunities for career advancement for minority nurses who were well established at MGH but without a way to progress.

A natural collaboration with Human Resources developed that resulted in nurse recruiters and members of the minority nurse committee attending the National Black Nurses Conventions, as well as job fairs at historically black colleges. To better reflect its work, the task force was renamed the Minority Nurse Retention and Recruitment Committee (MNRRC).

At MGH, the committee members made presentations to nursing administration and other key groups such as the Nursing Executive Committee. Support for the work of the committee continued to move forward under the leadership of Jeanette Ives Erickson, RN, MS, FAAN, senior vice president for Patient Care and chief nurse, when the hiring of minority nurses increased into the double digits.

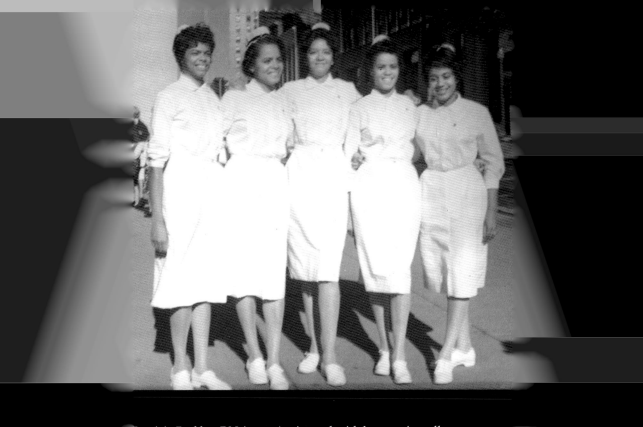

Patricia Beckles, RN (center), pictured with her cousins, all nurses, was a night nurse in MGH Pediatrics for 50 years and is still working per diem in 2011. According to hospital records, she has amassed the longest record

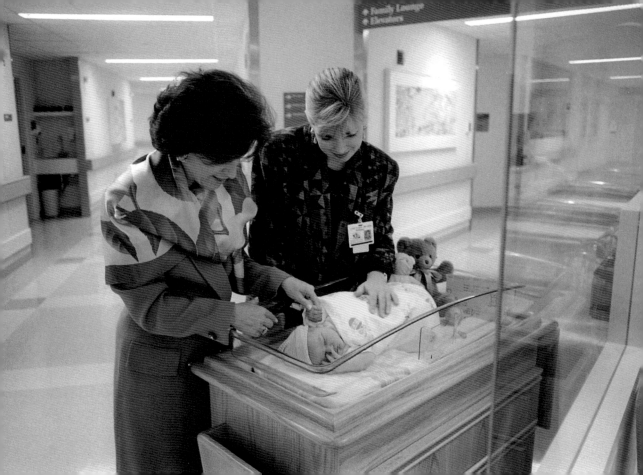

In the early 1990s, formal planning began for what would become the MGH Vincent Obstetrics Program. Among the many goals behind the move was to significantly improve the experience for trainees, as well as to provide vital continuity of care. This was particularly important for OB patients at the MGH community health centers, who would receive their prenatal care from MGH providers, and then have to deliver with an unfamiliar team at another hospital. How could MGH truly be a "general" hospital without obstetrics?

Obstetrics returned to MGH in 1994, under the leadership of Dr. Isaac Schiff, chief of Vincent Memorial Gynecology and Obstetrics, Dr. Fredric Frigoletto, Jr., chief of Obstetrics, and Jeanette Ives Erickson, RN, MS, FAAN, then director of both Obstetrics and Nursing Support Services. Members of the nursing leadership team were significant drivers of planning and implementation for the service, and recruited a team of skilled nurses and support staff that was critical to the program's success.

On July 5, MGH registered its first prenatal patient, and on November 2, the first delivery took place. The service was up, running and expanding rapidly. The Midwifery Program also formally began in 1994 with the hiring of the first nurse-midwife, Sherrin Langeler, CNM. She was soon joined by others, including Mary Eliot Jackson, CNM, the great-great-great granddaughter of MGH cofounder Dr. James Jackson. Today, the staff numbers 15 nurse-midwives, who are the attending providers for about one third of all deliveries at MGH. In 1997, the Division of Obstetrics and Gynecology was formally established. Most recently, the Vincent Obstetrics and Gynecology also extended its services to a suburban location, establishing a practice at MassGeneral West in Waltham, Mass. In 2011, the MGH Vincent Obstetrics Program will deliver its 50,000th baby.

Jeanette Ives Erickson, RN, MS, FAAN, senior vice president for Patient Care and chief nurse, was mentored by many nurse leaders. At Mercy Hospital in Portland, Maine, Sister Consuela, RN, and Eloise Paulin, RN, taught her the importance of strategic planning and sound budgeting. Muriel Poulin, professor at Boston University's School of Nursing, taught her

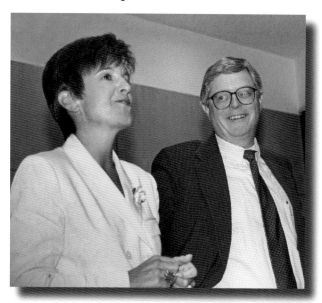

Pictured, Ives Erickson and Mongan

to position nursing to have a strong voice in the organization and about the importance of the integrity of the nurse-patient relationship. And Yvonne L. Munn, RN, inspired in her the importance of a robust nursing research program.

In the Fall of 1996, James J. Mongan, MD, president of the MGH, appointed Ives Erickson to lead Nursing and what had recently become Patient Care Services, in order to promote interdisciplinary collaboration. She immediately set about articulating a vision for the future. In collaboration with staff and leadership, she established the key components of a professional practice model, which included a clearly articulated vision, a staff-driven collaborative governance model, a clinical recognition advancement model, The Center for Clinical & Professional Development, a robust award and recognition program, and a narrative culture that brought the daily practice of clinicians to life through storytelling. She led the development of the Staff Perceptions of the Professional Practice Environment Survey, which provides clinicians with a formal mechanism to help evaluate and shape the practice environment.

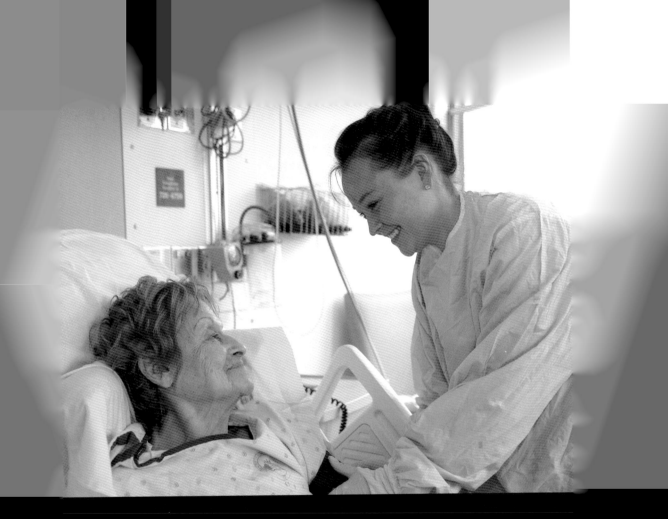

"If you keep your eye on the patient, you will always be headed in the right direction."

— Jeanette Ives Erickson, RN, MS, FAAN,
senior vice president for Patient Care and chief nurse

In 1996, Patient Care Services (PCS) began to cultivate a robust awards program to recognize excellence, beginning with the Stephanie M. Macaluso, RN, Excellence in Clinical Practice Award. Named in honor of Stephanie Macaluso, RN, thoracic clinical nurse specialist, the award was created to recognize clinicians whose practice was guided by critical thinking, mentoring, the ability to integrate knowledge, a focus on collaborative decision making and compassionate family-centered care — all attributes possessed by Macaluso.

Over the years, additional awards were created to recognize the contributions of nurses, including but not limited to the following:

- Norman Knight Preceptor of Distinction Award — recognizes a nurse who consistently demonstrates excellence in educating, precepting, coaching and mentoring other nurses.

- Brian M. McEachern Extraordinary Care Award — recognizes PCS staff whose passion and tenacity exceeds the expectations of patients, families and colleagues by demonstrating extraordinary acts of compassionate patient care and service.

- Jean M. Nardini, RN, Nurse Leader of Distinction Award — honors a staff nurse who demonstrates excellence in clinical practice and leadership and a commitment to the profession of nursing.

- Marie C. Petrilli Oncology Nursing Award — presented to an oncology nurse in recognition of his or her high level of caring, compassion and commitment as reflected in their care.

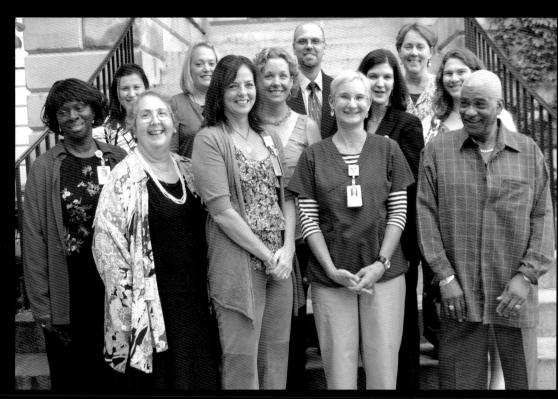

Pictured are the 2010 honorees at the inaugural Patient Care Services "One Celebration of Many Stars" event.

In 2010, Patient Care Services consolidated its recognition program into one annual award ceremony. On October 7, 2010, the first One Celebration of Many Stars ceremony was held on the Bulfinch Patio before a standing room-only crowd of staff, donors, patients and families.

In 1997, Collaborative Governance was established as a unique interdisciplinary model for communication and decision making in Patient Care Services.

Throughout its first decade, Collaborative Governance played an integral role in shaping and advancing the practice of the various disciplines comprising MGH Patient Care Services. The success of the program rested on its ability to shift clinical decision making from administrators to clinicians at the bedside. By empowering staff in this way, clinicians were positioned to use their knowledge, experience and commitment to provide the best possible care to patients and families. In 2011, collaborative governance was redesigned to ensure that it was aligned with current strategic, practice and quality initiatives.

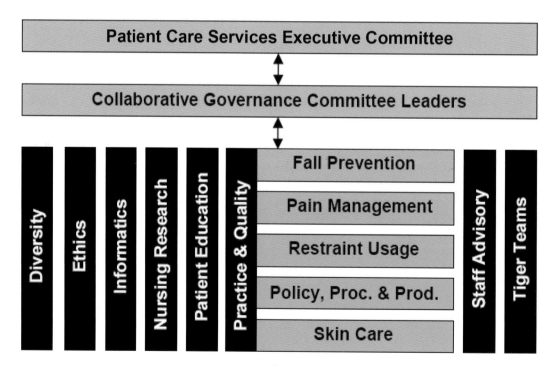

The 2010 redesigned Collaborative Governance model illustrates the various committees and subcommittees that have influence over the practice environment.

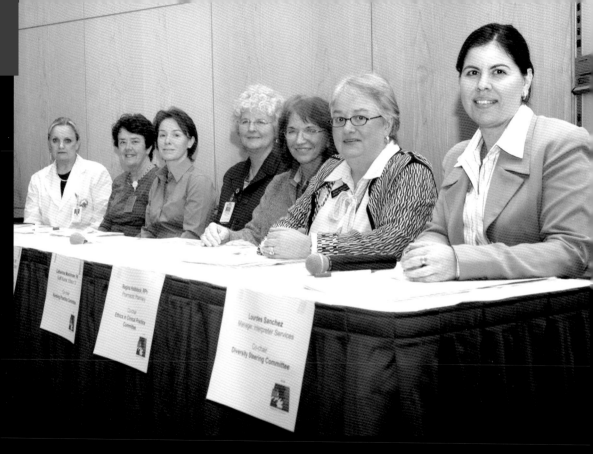

Representing their respective committees at the 2005 Collaborative Governance Annual Meeting are (l. to r.) Wendylee Baer, RN, Staff Nurse Advisory; Kathleen Tiberii, RN, Quality; Donna Lawson, RN, Patient Education; Catherine Griffith, RN, Research; Catherine MacKinaw, RN, Practice; Regina Holdstock, RPh, Ethics in Clinical Practice; and Lourdes Sanchez, MS, Diversity.

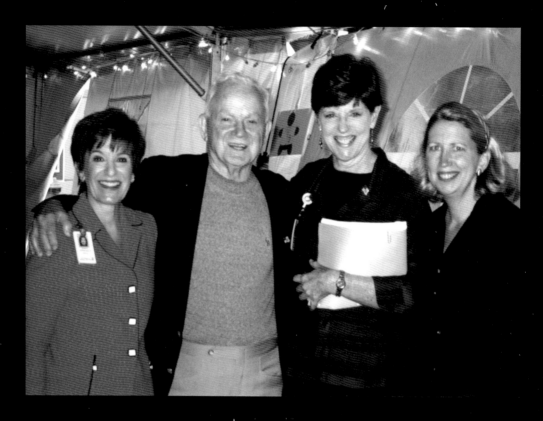

Pictured (l. to r.) are Jeanette Ives Erickson, RN, MS, FAAN; Norman Knight; Trish Gibbons, RN, DNSc, former associate chief nurse of The Norman Knight Nursing Center for Clinical & Professional Development; and Marianne Ditomassi, RN, MSN, MBA, first director of The Center for Clinical and Professional Development. With the 2007 dedication of The Norman Knight Nursing Center for Clinical & Professional Development, the state-of-the-art facility became one of the leading hospital-based nursing education centers in the country, featuring innovative orientation, training and continuing education programs; a variety of partnerships with academic institutions; clinical simulation training; the novel New Graduate Critical Care Nursing Program; and hundreds of continuing education programs designed to promote clinical excellence and professional development, including the Clinical Recognition Program, described at right.

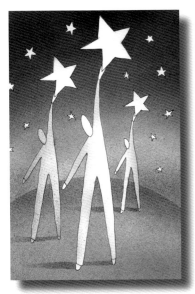

Clinicians in Patient Care Services at Massachusetts General Hospital have long valued their role in caring for patients and families. Created in 2002, the Clinical Recognition Program provides a way to formally recognize professional clinical staff for their expertise gained over time in the application of their discipline.

Based on the theoretical foundation of the Dreyfus Model of Skill Acquisition and the work of Patricia Benner, RN, PhD, FAAN, clinical staff from six Patient Care Services disciplines — nursing, occupational therapy, physical therapy, respiratory care, social work, and speech-language pathology — analyze their own practice through the themes and criteria of practice. Reflecting on the themes of clinician-patient relationship, clinical knowledge and decision making, teamwork and collaboration, and movement (for occupational therapy and physical therapy), and their identified criteria, clinicians can seek recognition for the level of practice they have achieved. The program was the first interdisciplinary recognition program in the country.

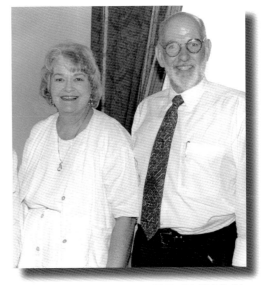

Patricia Benner, RN, PhD, FAAN (left), pictured with director emeritus Edward Coakley, RN, MEd, MA, MSN, visited the MGH in 1996 to discuss a narrative culture.

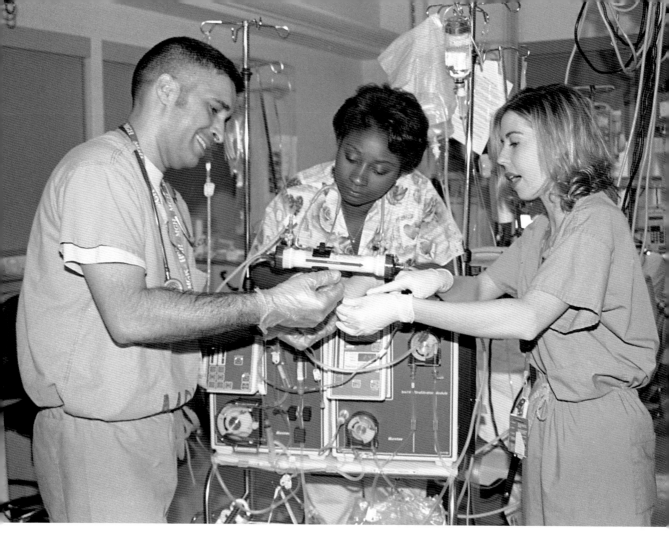

As the hospital continued to expand and diversify, so too did the population of patients served. It became clear that the staff needed to reflect these patients in order to best care for them. The 1997 Patient Care Services (PCS) strategic plan was designed to include a two-pronged approach to diversity: increase awareness and education around the delivery of culturally-competent care and develop meaningful efforts to increase the number of minorities in clinical and professional positions.

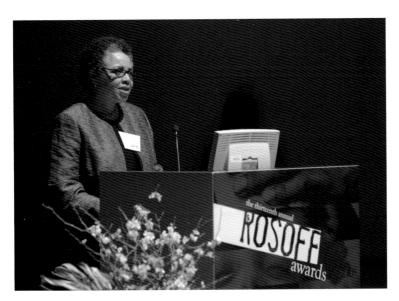

Deborah Washington, RN, PhD(c), accepting the inaugural Arnold Z. Rosoff "Agent of Change" Award

Deborah Washington, RN, PhD(c), became the first director of the newly formed PCS Diversity Program at a time when diversity was a relatively unfamiliar concept at MGH. She also became the first black leader to serve in MGH Nursing Administration. This move demonstrated to the community and to the country that MGH was serious about creating an environment where cultural diversity was an important part of health care. Through her leadership, diversity soon became an integral part of the PCS and hospital culture. By 2007, the number of minority nurses at MGH had doubled.

Various initiatives helped to promote diversity within the workforce, translate cultural competence into practice, and engage the MGH community in frank and direct conversation. A PCS Diversity Steering Committee was formed and charged with developing strategies to diversify the PCS workforce. Working with colleagues, Washington helped develop a culturally competent care curriculum offered monthly to staff. Multiple opportunities for MGH and the greater community to celebrate diversity were created, including an annual Diversity Holiday Fair and an African American Pinning Ceremony

diversity
MGH 1811
Patient Care Services

to formally recognize the contributions of African American colleagues. The Hausman Student Nurse Fellowship was established to provide students with a rare opportunity to work with a minority mentor while developing essential skill sets needed to thrive in the workplace.

The impact of the program and the influence of its director extended well beyond the walls of the MGH. Various components of the program were and continue to be replicated at health care organizations throughout the country. And, among other notable honors, Washington gained regional recognition when the Arnold Z. Rosoff "Agent of Change" Award was established to recognize the scope and impact of her work.

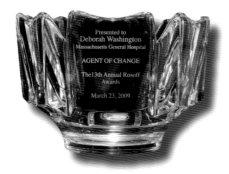

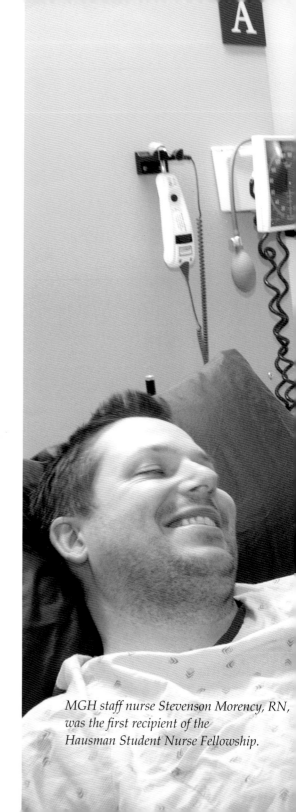

MGH staff nurse Stevenson Morency, RN, was the first recipient of the Hausman Student Nurse Fellowship.

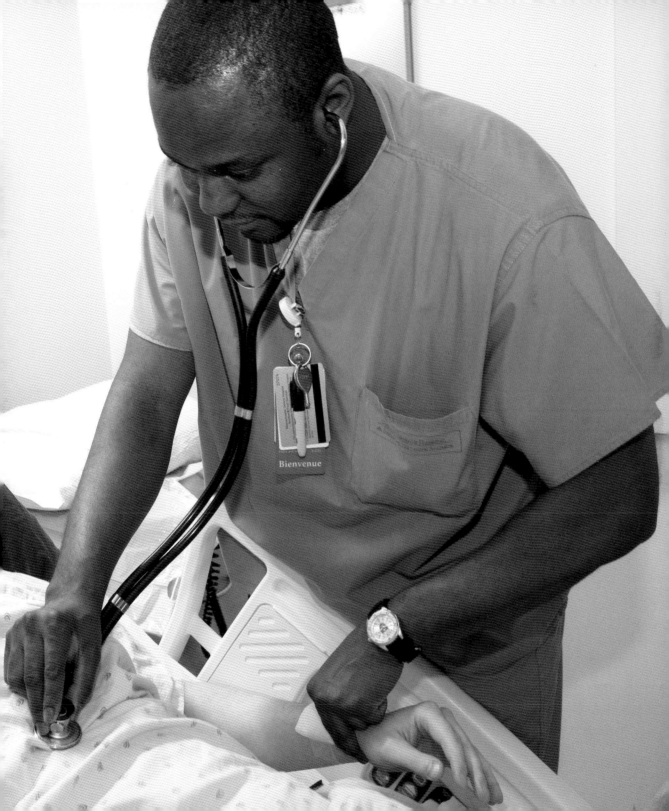

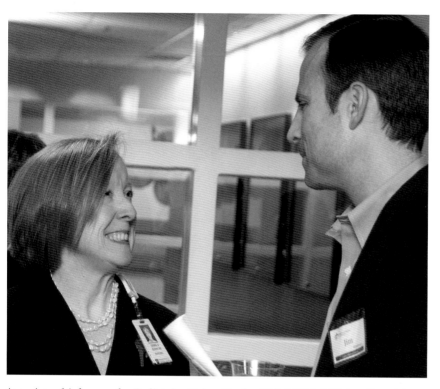

Associate chief nurse for Pediatrics Debra Burke, RN, MSN, MBA, talks with MassGeneral Hospital for *Children PFAC member Jim Massman.*

In 1999, MGH established its first patient and family advisory council (PFAC) within the MassGeneral Hospital *for* Children. The goal was to encourage patients and families to directly influence hospital decision making and care delivery. MGH has since formed two additional clinically based PFACs — co-led by a patient or family member and a nurse — within the Cancer Center (2001) and the Heart Center (2007).

PFACs are grounded in the belief that often the most informed voices on the care team are those of the patient and family. Ultimately, they alone can confirm whether a plan of care was explained thoroughly; the clinical information provided was fully understood; their questions and fears were appropriately addressed; care was tailored to their specific needs; they felt safe; systems worked efficiently and effectively; and each was treated as a whole person.

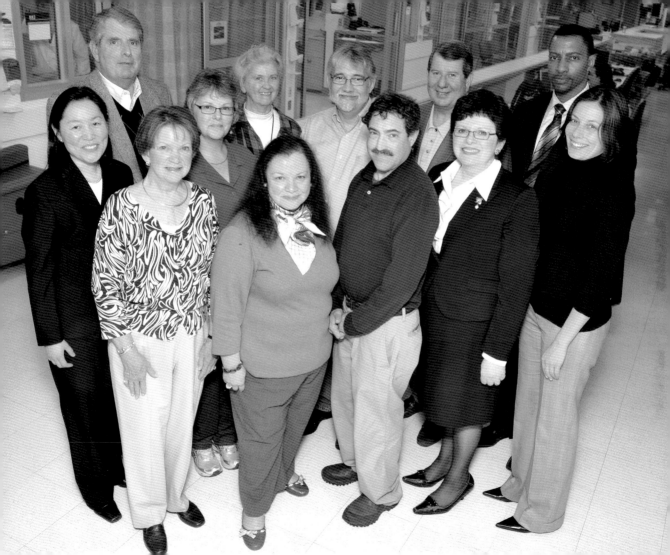

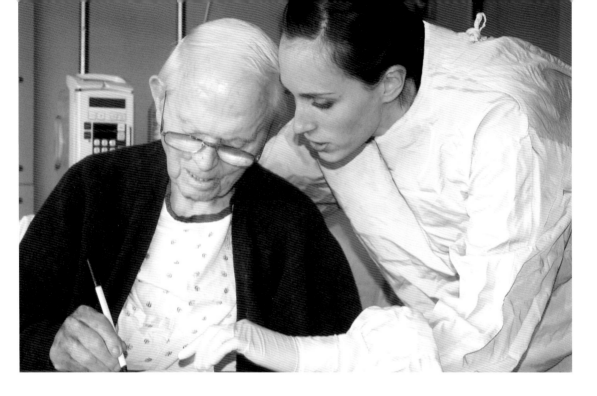

Reports released after the year 2000 began to indicate that by 2030, the number of people over the age of 62 would double, from 40 million to 80 million. This would place an unprecedented demand on the health care system. In anticipation, tailoring

In 2007, veteran MGH nurse Ed Coakley, RN, received a major grant from the Health Resources and Services Administration to fund the innovative RN Residency Program: Transitioning to Geriatrics and Palliative Care.

The RN Residency Program was

nursing experience receive advanced education in geriatrics and palliative care. A complementary four-month Preceptor Program for RNs age 45 and older provides similar specialty education, grooming them to serve as clinical preceptors or mentors for the nurse residents.

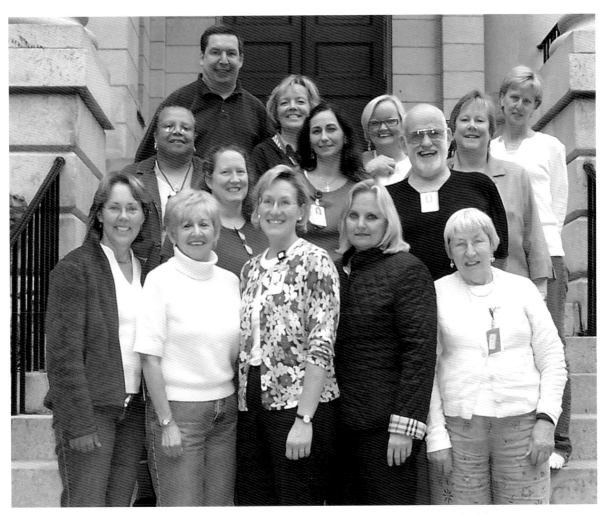

Ed Coakley, RN, director emeritus, (second row, far right), pictured with the first group of geropalliative care nurse residents.

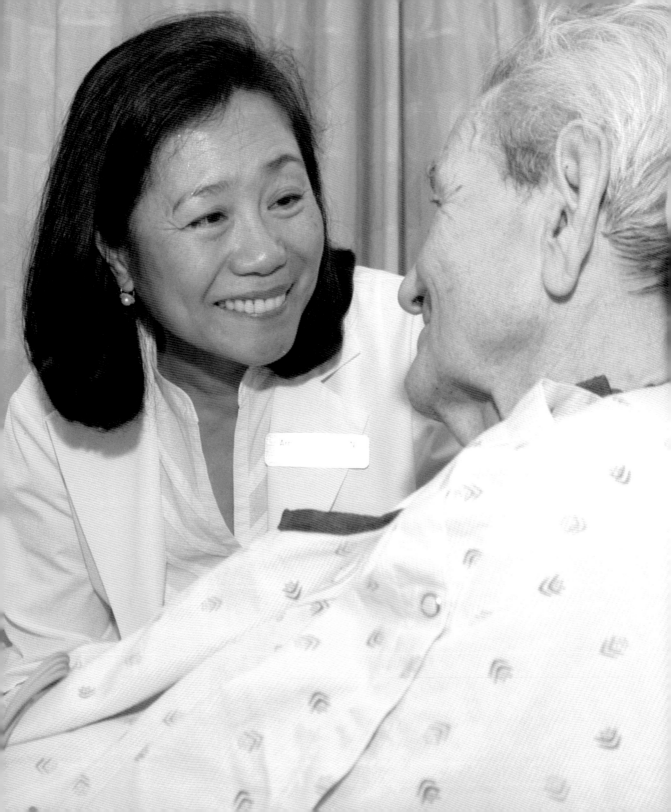

Based on a curriculum developed by New York University School of Education called NICHE (Nurses Improving Care for Health System Elders), under the leadership of Deborah D'Avolio, RN, PhD, MGH launched its own 65*plus* program. This highly specialized, interdisciplinary model of care was designed to focus on meeting the needs of older patients by providing unit-based education, support for geriatric certification, annual conferences to share best practices and more. 65*plus* began to systematically add to the knowledge and skill base of MGH nurses and other clinicians.

In 2010, the Center to Champion Nursing in America, a joint venture of the AARP and the Robert Wood Johnson Foundation, cosponsored ageWISE, a program designed to disseminate nationally the lessons learned in the RN Residency Program. In the first phase, six geographically distributed U.S. hospitals — required to be both NICHE and Magnet designated hospitals — were selected to test the program on a variety of institutional contexts.

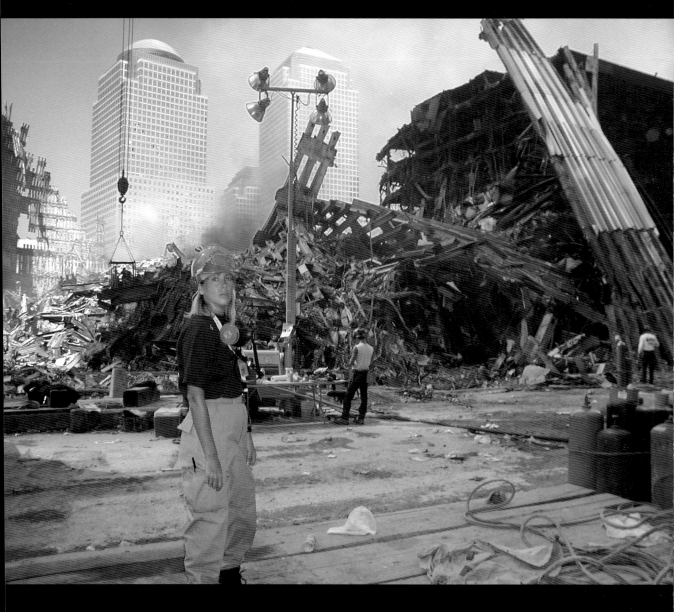

Brenda Smith, RN, NP, an MGH IMSuRT team member, provided care to workers at Ground Zero out of a deli the team had converted into a medical station. Here she pauses in front of the rubble on her way to pick up supplies. To the far left is the site of a fire station that lost all of its members in the terrorist attack; the domed towers are the American Express building; and in the foreground is the location of the former Marriott Hotel and Tower Three.

On the morning of September 11, 2001, terrorists crashed commercial airliners into the Twin Towers in New York City; the Pentagon in Washington, D.C.; and a field in Pennsylvania, claiming nearly 3,000 lives, injuring hundreds, and leaving an entire country confused and in mourning. In its first-ever deployment, the MGH-based International Medical Surgical Response Team (IMSuRT), along with the Metro Boston Disaster Medical Assistance Team (DMAT), arrived at Ground Zero on the evening of September 13. Shortly before, a building had collapsed on the site initially chosen for their medical station. Throughout a cold and rainy night, the team set up the first of what would be five medical stations, and by 7 a.m. they were seeing patients. MGH IMSuRT and the other Boston disaster teams went on to treat more than 5,000 workers during the first 11 days following the disaster.

In 2002, the nursing profession was facing a serious and worsening nursing shortage. Recognizing that the general public did not have an accurate picture of nursing, MGH Nursing began to aggressively work to change this through a variety of efforts, including an ad campaign that featured a diversity of MGH nurses, a hugely successful Employee Referral Program, several nursing expos and media outreach. The goal was to recruit the best and brightest by making the pride and passion MGH nurses felt for their profession known by having MGH nurses tell the MGH story.

MGH Nursing was featured in the first of a 2004 three-part documentary series titled *Lifeline: Nursing Diaries,* which aired on the Discovery Health Channel. Creator, videographer and producer Richard Kahn and his team spent months shadowing MGH nurses on the hospital's Cardiac Surgical, Neonatal and Surgical intensive care units. The final hour of television provided an authentic glimpse of bedside nursing that the Center for Nursing Advocacy described as "possibly the best single hour of a nursing documentary" they had ever seen.

Early in 2005, the MGH Department of Nursing pitched a story idea to reporter Scott Allen at *The Boston Globe:* shadow an experienced and a new graduate nurse dyad in an ICU for several months to help educate the public about "today's nurse." The result was a four-part, front page series "Critical Care: The making of an ICU nurse"and a companion multimedia website. The series was lauded for giving "readers an unusually vivid sense of the complexity and importance of highly

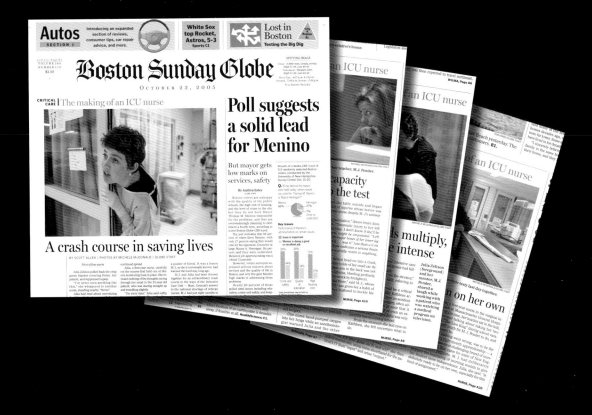

skilled nursing in a major hospital, with some indication of the stress the nursing crisis has put on critical health systems." MGH Nursing reprinted and distributed the articles to high school science teachers and nursing schools nationwide as a way of recruiting and retaining the next generation of nurses, and the series became a formal part of the curriculum of several noteworthy nursing programs. The initiative received national and international acclaim from a variety of professional organizations, including the American Academy of Nursing and Sigma Theta Tau International.

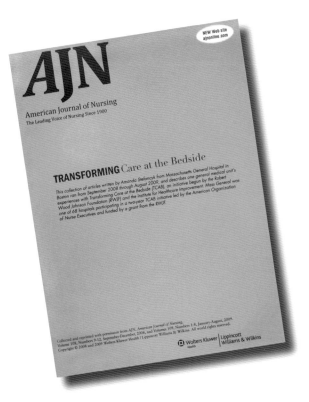

This collection of articles written by Amanda Stefancyk from Massachusetts General Hospital in Boston ran from September 2008 through August 2009, and describes one general medical unit's experiences with Transforming Care at the Bedside (TCAB), an initiative begun by the Robert Wood Johnson Foundation (RWJF) and the Institute for Healthcare Improvement. Mass General was one of 68 hospitals participating in a two-year TCAB initiative led by the American Organization of Nurse Executives and funded by a grant from the RWJF.

Image of reprint cover used with permission.
Copyright American Journal of Nursing.
All rights reserved.

Beginning in September of 2008, Amanda Stefancyk, RN, MSN, MBA, nursing director of the White 10 General Medical Unit, authored her first in a yearlong series of articles published in the *American Journal of Nursing (AJN).* The series chronicled her unit's experience participating in the two-year Transforming Care at the Bedside (TCAB) project to improve patient care and enhance the retention of nurses. Jointly sponsored by the Robert Wood Johnson Foundation, Institute for Healthcare Improvement, and American Organization of Nurse Executives, TCAB was a national program designed to engage nurses as leaders, providing them with tools and training to drive improvements in the quality and safety of patient care delivery on medical and surgical units. MGH was the only full-service academic medical center in Massachusetts to participate.

Pictured (at right) is Mike O'Donnell, RN, MGH Emergency Department, one of many MGH staff members who appeared in the eight-part ABC series Boston Med.

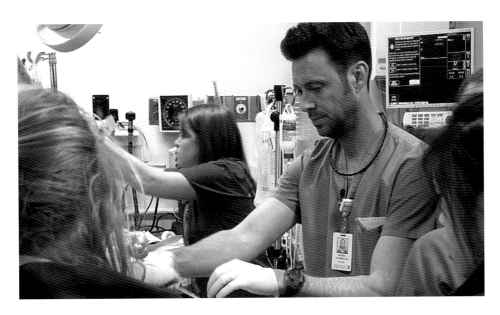

BOSTONMED

A Real Life Medical Drama
from America's Top Hospitals

In 2010, MGH Nursing was once again featured in a nationally broadcast ABC series called *Boston Med*. The eight-hour series provided an in-depth look behind the scenes at MGH and two other Boston hospitals by following individual providers and patients. MGH nurses were among those prominently featured.

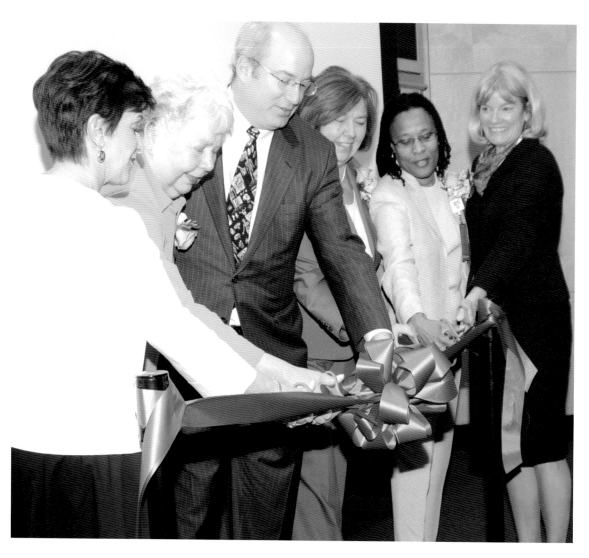

A special ceremony was held in 2008 to formally dedicate The Yvonne L. Munn Center for Nursing Research (located on the fourth floor of the Professional Office Building on Cambridge Street). Pictured above (l. to r.) are Jeanette Ives Erickson, RN, MS, FAAN; Yvonne L. Munn, RN; MGH president, Peter Slavin, MD; director of the Munn Center, Dorothy Jones, RNC, EdD, FAAN; executive director of The Institute for Patient Care, Gaurdia Banister, RN, PhD; and special guest speaker, Terry Fulmer, RN, PhD, FAAN, national nursing leader and researcher.

"Develop a spirit of inquiry. If you begin to ask questions about your own practice, on every aspect of it, and you don't like the answer on some of those, then study it and change it. That's what research is."

— *Yvonne L. Munn, RN, MS,*
associate general director and
director of Nursing, 1984-1993

In 2003, MGH formalized several research activities under the auspices of a dedicated research center named for and endowed by Yvonne L. Munn, RN, associate general director and director of Nursing at MGH from 1984 to 1993.

The Munn Center supports a growing inventory of research-related programs and activities, including a postdoctoral nursing fellowship program; a peer-support and networking group for doctorally prepared staff, now numbering more than 30; a grant program for clinical staff interested in conducting research within a practice setting under the mentorship of a doctorally prepared nurse scientist; and a nurse-scientist advancement model.

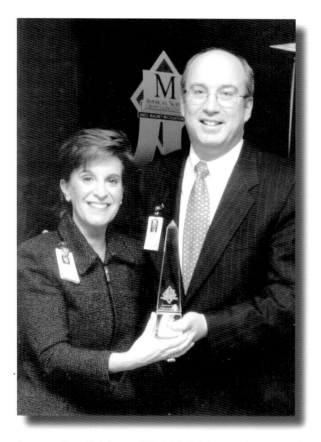

Jeanette Ives Erickson, RN, MS, FAAN, and MGH president Peter L. Slavin, MD, MBA, are pictured with the Magnet Award.

On September 4, 2003, seven years after launching the professional practice model for Nursing and Patient Care Services, MGH became the only hospital in Massachusetts to be Magnet designated. This is the highest honor bestowed on a health care organization by the American Nurses Credentialing Center for excellence in nursing services. The formal recognition program began in the late 1990s, and MGH became only the 83rd hospital to receive the honor, earned by only 1 percent of all hospitals in the country at that time. In 2007, MGH was redesignated through 2012.

The Magnet Recognition Program is grounded in research study titled "Magnet Hospitals: Attraction and Retention of Professional Nurses." The study was conducted in 1983 by Margaret L. McClure, EdD, RN, FAAN; Muriel A. Poulin, EdD, RN, FAAN, MGH School of Nursing, class of 1946; Margaret D. Sovie, PhD, FAAN, CRNP; and Mabel A. Wandelt, RN, PhD, at the request of the American Academy of Nursing (AAN).

The AAN Task Force on Nursing Practice in Hospitals studied 163 hospitals to identify and describe variables that created an environment that attracted and retained well-qualified nurses who promoted quality patient/resident/client care. Forty-one of the 163 institutions were described as "Magnet" hospitals because of their ability to attract and retain professional nurses. The characteristics that seem to distinguish "Magnet" organizations from others became known as the "Forces of Magnetism."

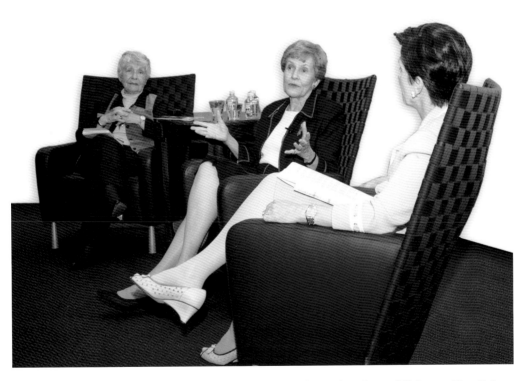

Muriel Poulin, RN (left), and Margaret McClure, RN, (center) authors of "Magnet Hospitals: Attraction and Retention of Professional Nurses," the original Magnet hospital study conducted in 1983, were featured guests during MGH Nurse Recognition Week in 2008.

"As I escorted the Magnet appraiser throughout MGH, I couldn't have been more impressed or more proud."

— *Joanne Parhiala, RN, MGH staff nurse and Magnet
ambassador, a liaison with the Magnet champions*

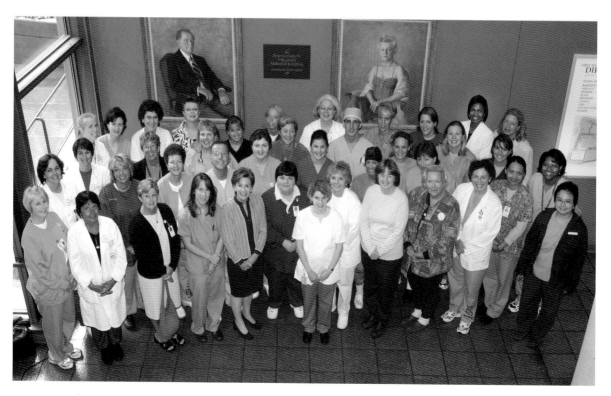

Above, the MGH's first group of Magnet champions

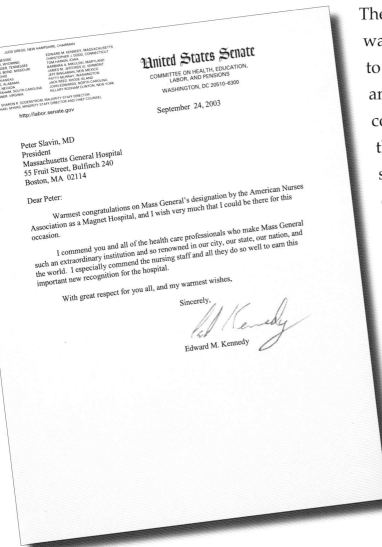

United States Senate

COMMITTEE ON HEALTH, EDUCATION,
LABOR, AND PENSIONS

WASHINGTON, DC 20510–6300

September 24, 2003

Peter Slavin, MD
President
Massachusetts General Hospital
55 Fruit Street, Bulfinch 240
Boston, MA 02114

Dear Peter:

Warmest congratulations on Mass General's designation by the American Nurses Association as a Magnet Hospital, and I wish very much that I could be there for this occasion.

I commend you and all of the health care professionals who make Mass General such an extraordinary institution and so renowned in our city, our state, our nation, and the world. I especially commend the nursing staff and all they do so well to earn this important new recognition for the hospital.

With great respect for you all, and my warmest wishes,

Sincerely,

Edward M. Kennedy

The Magnet champion role was designed for staff nurses to discover, communicate and motivate the MGH community to prepare for the Magnet recognition site visit. The staff nurse champion role was subsequently utilized to promote other key Patient Care Services and hospitalwide initiatives, such as Joint Commission readiness, which, under the leadership of Keith Perleberg, RN, MDiv, mobilized Excellence Every Day champions.

U.S. Senator Edward M. Kennedy sent his congratulations upon learning of the hospital's Magnet designation, stating, in part, "I commend you and all of the health care professionals who make Mass General such an extraordinary institution ... I especially commend the nursing staff for all they do so well..."

In 2004, Grace Deveney, RN, BSN, MPH, and Katie Fallon, RN, BSN, were the first nurses awarded a Thomas S. Durant Fellowship for Refugee Medicine. The program honors the spirit of Thomas S. Durant, MD, former MGH associate general director, who throughout his life incorporated humanitarian service to refugees, victims both of war and of natural disasters, into his professional practice.

The two spent six months caring for victims of a bloody conflict in the Darfur region of Sudan, which United Nations officials described as the world's worst humanitarian crisis. More than one million people were forced to flee their homes and turn to refugee camps for survival.

Deveney worked with a nutrition team in El Geniena in northwestern Darfur, helping train local staff in the operation and management of community-based therapeutic care (CTC). Fallon became involved in establishing a primary health clinic in Donki Dreissa, which lies along a village-dotted corridor between Nyala and Girayda, an area that was considered "unsecured."

Since then, six more MGH nurses have been awarded Durant Fellowships: Lucinda Langenkamp, RN, APRN, BC (2006), worked in Rwanda on HIV prevention, care and treatment; Chanda Plong, RN (2006), provided surgical services throughout Southeast Asia; Betsy Deitte, RN, BSN (2008), traveled to Zambia to help reduce maternal and infant mortality associated with childbirth; Heather Szymczak, RN, BSN (2008), provided care to the underserved in Central America; Jennifer Brock, RN (2008), provided palliative and HIV care and studied TB in South Africa; and Joy Williams, RN, BSN (2010), provided care in a clinic in Haiti in the weeks and months following a devastating earthquake.

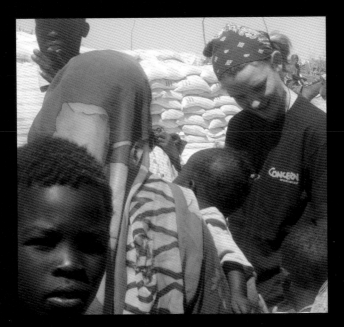

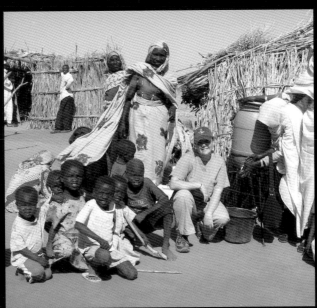

*Grace Deveney, RN, BSN, MPH (top), and Katie Fallon,
RN, BSN (bottom), spent six months in the Darfur region of
Sudan providing care to victims of a violent civil war.*

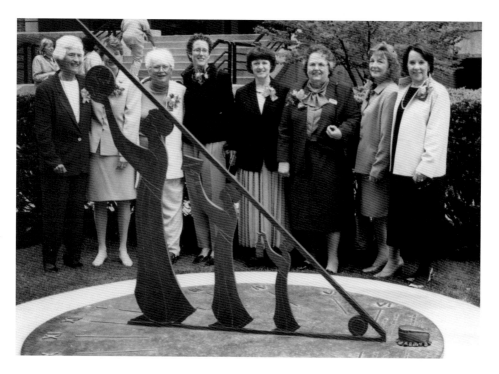

Pictured at the dedication of the MGH Nursing Sundial is sculptor Nancy Schön (far left) with members of the MGH Nurses' Alumnae Association.

During Nurse Recognition Week 2004, a crowd of MGH staff, employees, volunteers and friends joined members of the MGH Nurses' Alumnae Association in the formal unveiling of a permanent tribute to MGH Nursing — the MGH Nursing Sundial. Sculpted by Nancy Schön, best known for her Make Way for Ducklings installment in Boston's Public Garden, the sculpture acknowledges the important contributions and critical thinking of nurses within the field of health care. Schön also wanted the finished design to attract future generations of nurses. The sculpture was a gift of the MGH Nurses' Alumnae Association.

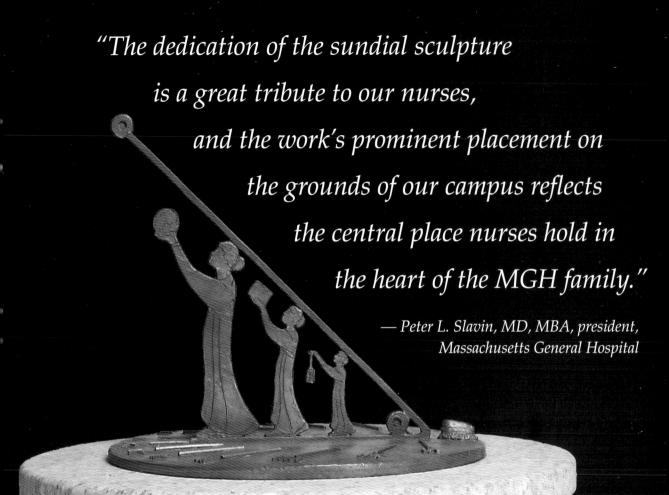

*"The dedication of the sundial sculpture
is a great tribute to our nurses,
and the work's prominent placement on
the grounds of our campus reflects
the central place nurses hold in
the heart of the MGH family."*

— *Peter L. Slavin, MD, MBA, president,
Massachusetts General Hospital*

*The figures of the MGH Nursing Sundial sculpture depict the profession's past
and a tribute to Florence Nightingale (holding a lantern, charting the course for the
profession); present (holding a book, representing the scientific knowledge base for the
profession); and future (holding a globe, representing the far-reaching, global impact of
nursing and its universal and multicultural dimensions).*

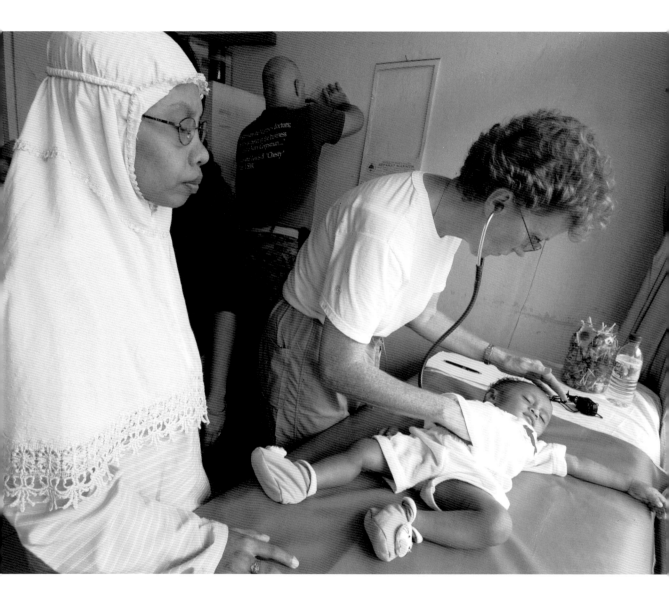

MGH staff nurse Karen Holland, RN, volunteered with Project HOPE as part of the Military Sealift Command (MSC) hospital ship USNS **Mercy** *(T-AH 19). Here she examines an Indonesian child at the Kalabahi Hospital in Alor, Indonesia.*

2005 began in dramatic fashion just after a devastating tsunami hit the coast of Indonesia. Tens of thousands perished, and countless more were left injured and suffering. The United States pledged its help to these victims, and more than 75 MGH clinicians answered the call. Shortly after the new year began, the first wave of MGH staff stepped aboard the recommissioned U.S. Naval Ship *Mercy*, anchored two miles off the coast of Banda Aceh as part of a relief effort organized by Project HOPE. This was the first time in history the U.S. government had allowed civilian health care providers to work alongside their military colleagues.

The pilot program proved a huge success and, just months later, was replicated closer to home when Hurricanes Katrina and Rita left more than a million people along the U.S. Gulf Coast homeless and/ or displaced. Again, the MGH community answered a call from Project HOPE to provide aid to area victims. Many other MGH staff went to the Gulf Coast with the U.S. Public Health Service and the Massachusetts Disaster Medical Assistance Team. Dozens and dozens of MGH volunteers stepped forward to help, and countless clinicians lined up to provide the coverage needed during their colleagues' absence.

Karen Holland, RN, a staff nurse in the Emergency Department and prior volunteer on the USNS *Mercy*, served as chief nursing officer aboard the USNS *Comfort*, where she oversaw all Project HOPE nursing volunteers aboard the ship.

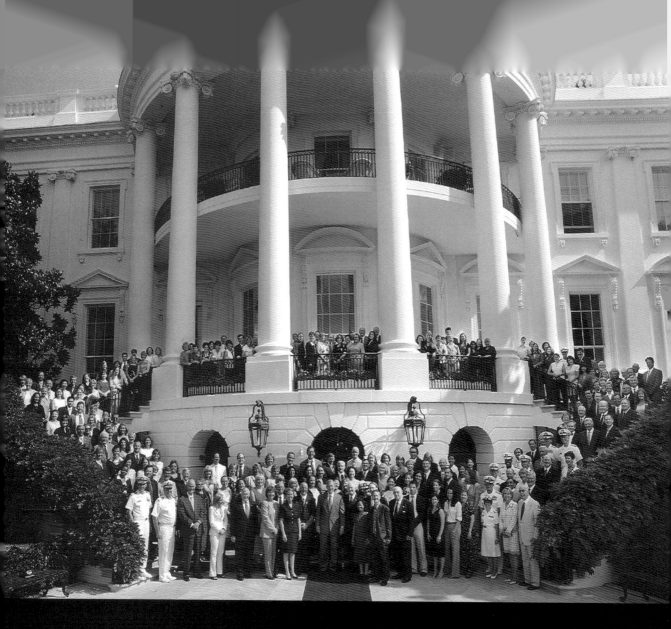

At a formal ceremony on the South Lawn of the White House, President George W. Bush honored the Project HOPE disaster relief team, which included nearly 100 MGH clinical volunteers — all of whom assisted in post-tsunami relief efforts. The Project HOPE volunteers, along with the U.S. Navy's Operation Unified Assistance, evaluated and treated more than 49,500 patients and performed more than 97,000 medical procedures onshore and aboard the

HONORING THE MASSACHUSETTS GENERAL HOSPITAL

Mr. President, I join with President Bush and Project HOPE in commending the extraordinary work of the health professionals from Massachusetts General Hospital who dropped everything and went to Indonesia in January and February to provide medical care to survivors of the tsunami disaster. I especially commend Dr. Laurence Ronan, the group leader at MGH who did so much to organize the trip.

These dedicated health professionals answered the urgent call when disaster struck. As in the past when earthquakes devastated Armenia, and El Salvador, and Iran, they volunteered their services and skills on the USNS *Mercy*, the Navy hospital ship sent to the coast of Indonesia.

Massachusetts General Hospital sent the largest health team. More than 60 doctors, nurses and social workers each spent a month helping on cases too complex to be treated by personnel already on the ground in Indonesia. They had expertise in critical medical specialties such as neurology, burns, lung disease, kidney disease, and pediatrics, and they provided care to hundreds devastated by the tsunami.

Massachusetts is very proud of MGH and the extraordinary health professionals being honored today. Their dedication and caring have served America and the world well."

— Senator Edward M. Kennedy
Congressional Record, *July 21, 2005*

Jean M. Nardini, RN Hemodialysis Unit

In April of 2006, the MGH community formally dedicated the Jean M. Nardini, RN, Hemodialysis Unit, the first MGH patient care unit named in honor of a nurse. Nardini's sphere of influence was far-reaching. Her MGH career spanned nearly four decades, marked by a legacy of innovation and progressive thinking, a quick wit and hands-on leadership style. She entered hemodialysis nursing in 1969 when the specialty was in its infancy, and went on to become a nationally recognized expert in the care of patients on hemodialysis, serving as president of the American Nephrology Nurses' Association. When she died in 2005, following a long battle with cancer, Nardini was nurse manager of the Hemodialysis Unit, a position held for nearly 30 years. In her lifetime, she taught countless nurses, physicians and fellows, and was widely published.

Nardini became the first recipient of the Jean M. Nardini, RN, Nurse of Distinction Award, established in her honor just prior to her death. Thereafter presented annually, the award recognizes a nurse who consistently demonstrates excellence in clinical practice, leadership, and patient- and family-centered care, as well as a dedication to the nursing profession.

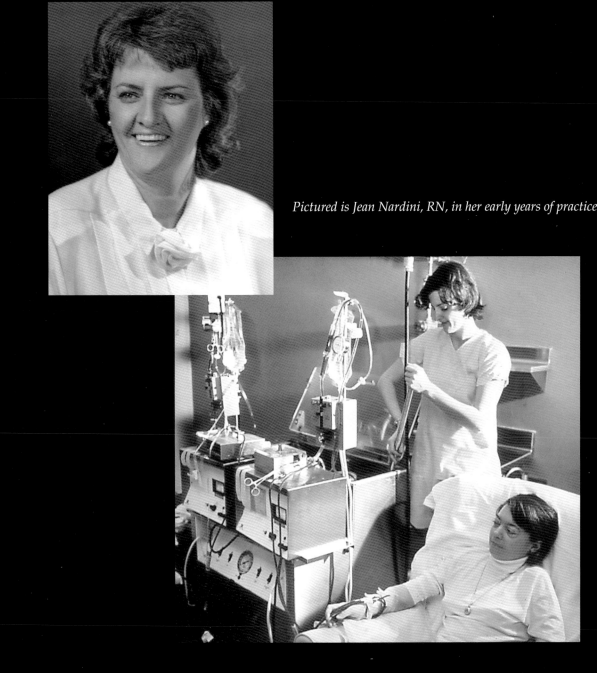

Pictured is Jean Nardini, RN, in her early years of practice

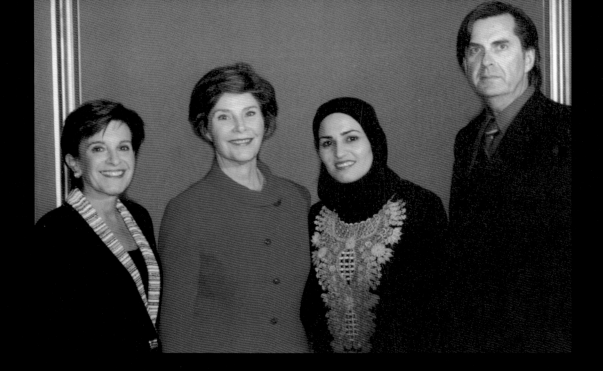

ABOVE: In October of 2005, Project HOPE hosted a dinner at the Mellon Auditorium in Washington, D.C., to benefit the creation of the Basrah Children's Hospital of Iraq. First Lady Laura Bush and U.S. Secretary of State Condoleezza Rice addressed the crowd. Pictured at the event are (l. to r.) Jeanette Ives Erickson, RN, MS, FAAN, senior vice president for Patient Care and chief nurse; First Lady Laura Bush; Sukaina Matter, RN, chief nurse, Basrah Children's Hospital; and Fred Gerber, Project HOPE, country director, Iraq and Special Projects.

BELOW: Basrah Children's Hospital under construction.

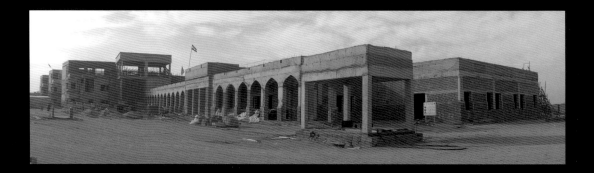

MGH became very involved in 2006 with a major venture in Iraq. Working with Project HOPE and the U.S. Agency for International Development, Jeanette Ives Erickson, RN, MS, FAAN, senior vice president for Patient Care and chief nurse, served as senior nurse consultant on an initiative to build and staff a pediatric oncology hospital — Basrah Children's Hospital in southern Iraq. She became responsible for mentoring the hospital's chief nurse, Sukaina Matter, RN, and for ensuring that the hospital's Iraqi nurses were appropriately trained and prepared to provide high-quality, specialized care to children. This work was also supported by the nurses within the MassGeneral Hospital *for* Children and MGH Medical Interpreter Services.

In 2006, Ives Erickson also visited the King Abdullah Hospital in Jordan and the Royal Hospital of Muscat in Oman, where more than 200 nurses were being trained for their upcoming Basrah assignments. She had an opportunity to review the curriculum, talk with Iraqi nurses, exchange thoughts and ideas, and get a sense of the progress being made in preparing these nurses to practice in oncology nursing.

Patient Care Services (PCS) assumed a bold agenda for shaping the future delivery of patient care with the 2006 launch of The Institute for Patient Care. The Institute represents a first-of-its-kind interdisciplinary initiative, designed to bring together all disciplines to creatively innovate and generate new ideas to advance a core mission of patient care, education and research. The Institute supports collaboration between well-established PCS programs and centers — The Norman Knight Nursing Center for Clinical & Professional Development, The Yvonne L. Munn Center for Nursing Research, and The Maxwell & Eleanor Blum Patient and Family Learning Center, a nurse-led patient and family service that opened in 1999 to provide important health information to the public. The Center for Innovations

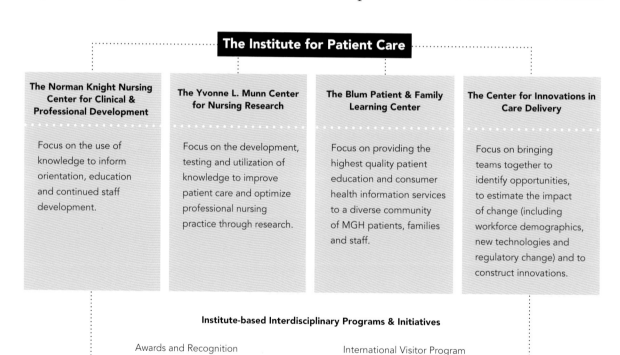

The Institute for Patient Care

The Norman Knight Nursing Center for Clinical & Professional Development	The Yvonne L. Munn Center for Nursing Research	The Blum Patient & Family Learning Center	The Center for Innovations in Care Delivery
Focus on the use of knowledge to inform orientation, education and continued staff development.	Focus on the development, testing and utilization of knowledge to improve patient care and optimize professional nursing practice through research.	Focus on providing the highest quality patient education and consumer health information services to a diverse community of MGH patients, families and staff.	Focus on bringing teams together to identify opportunities, to estimate the impact of change (including workforce demographics, new technologies and regulatory change) and to construct innovations.

Institute-based Interdisciplinary Programs & Initiatives

Awards and Recognition
Clinical Recognition Program
Collaborative Governance
Consultation
Culturally Competent Care
Ethics and Clinical Decision-Making

International Visitor Program
Leadership Development
Organizational Evaluation
Simulation Training
Workforce Development

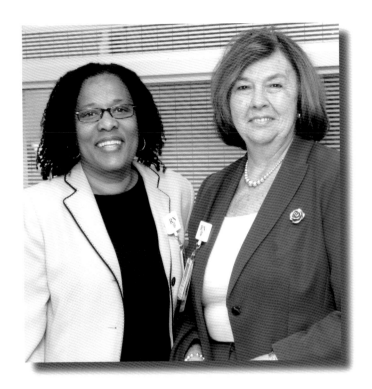

Pictured (l. to r.) are Gaurdia Banister, RN, PhD, the first executive director of The Institute for Patient Care, and Dorothy Jones, RNC, EdD, FAAN, the first director of The Yvonne L. Munn Center for Nursing Research.

in Care Delivery opened in 2006 to bring teams together to identify opportunities, to estimate the impact of change, and to construct innovation in care delivery. The Institute's "next generation" infrastructure is strategically designed to foster teamwork; share best practices; and bring an informed, interdisciplinary approach to patient- and family-centered care.

The formation of the Institute capped a decade of work that had become an integral part the interdisciplinary PCS culture, including the development of a vibrant professional practice model, formation of a robust structure for collaborative decision making, delivery of cutting-edge professional development programs, establishment of a multimedia learning center for patients and families, and formalization of a comprehensive nursing research program.

Formally dedicated in June of 2007, The Norman Knight Nursing Center for Clinical & Professional Development was built on the work of its first director, Marianne Ditomassi, RN, MSN, MBA, that shifted the focus of nursing education from training and development to "continuous learning."

Today, led by Gino Chisari, RN, MSN, the Norman Knight Nursing Center supports a robust array of professional development activities, including orientation, continuing education and simulation, affiliations with schools of nursing and leadership development programs, and education-related consultation locally, nationally and internationally.

Former president of RKO Radio, Norman Knight had a successful career in broadcasting. A prominent philanthropist, in 1959 he founded The Hundred Club of Massachusetts, which benefits more than 60,000 police officers and firefighters and their family members, totaling more than 250,000 individuals.

At the time, Knight's $1 million donation marked the largest gift ever received by the MGH Department of Nursing.

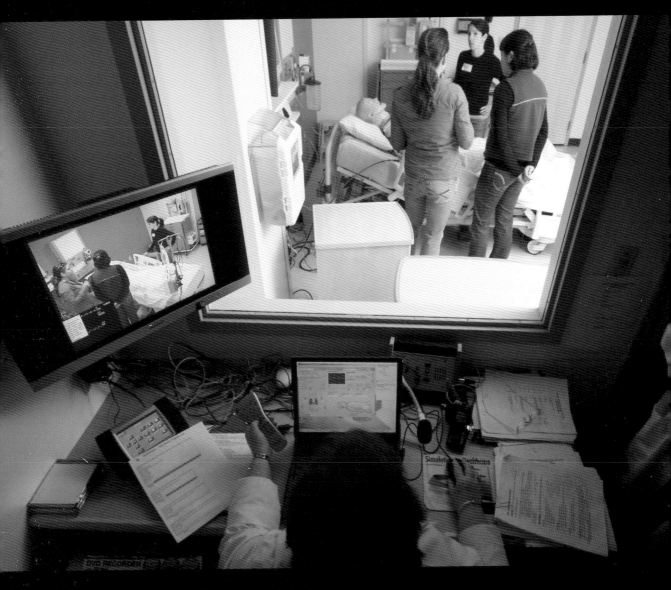

In 2006, Patient Care Services opened two new state-of-the-art simulation training sites, one in The Norman Knight Nursing Center for Clinical & Professional Development and the other strategically located adjacent to the PCS Office of Quality and Safety, The Yvonne L. Munn Nursing Research Center and The Center for Innovations in Care Delivery. Each simulation site features lifelike mannequins that can be computer operated to emit vocal sounds, breathing sounds and cardiac rhythms that mimic particular medical events, such as a sudden drop in blood pressure or a heart attack.

In an effort to promote the delivery of high-quality care and advance the nursing profession, MGH Nursing has been privileged to partner with nursing services around the world, including hospitals in Dubai, Iraq, Bermuda, and, most recently, China. Using a twinning model, a flexible framework to help organizations learn and master clinical skills, MGH Nursing provides peer-to-peer exchange and expert consultation to achieve these goals.

The International Nurse Consultant Program was developed in 1995. This program provides an opportunity for nurses from all over the globe to come to MGH and consult with expert nurse leaders and clinicians. From 2005 through 2010, MGH Nursing hosted 440 visitors representing 23 different countries, including Argentina, Australia, China, Greece, Israel, Japan, Kenya, Northern Ireland, South Korea and Thailand.

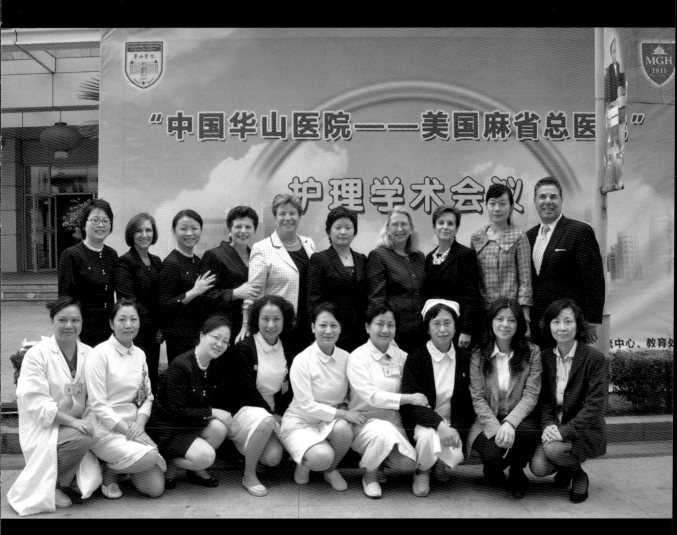

Pictured with members of the nursing staff at Huashan Hospital in Shanghai, China, during a 2010 visit are (back row, second from left) Colleen Snydeman, RN, MSN; (fourth and fifth from left) Theresa Gallivan, RN, MS; Dawn Tenney, RN, MSN; (seventh and eight from left) Marianne Ditomassi, RN, MSN, MBA; Jeanette Ives Erickson, RN, MS, FAAN; and (far right) Gino Chisari, RN, MSN. The sign behind them reads "Huashan Hospital of China and Mass General Hospital of United States: Nursing Care Seminar."

In 2010, the eyes of the world focused on the tiny nation of Haiti, after a 7.0 magnitude earthquake left thousands dead and thousands more seriously injured. The country's infrastructure, particularly its health care system, completely collapsed. Once again, MGH led the nation, by immediately committing staff to provide humanitarian relief, the majority of whom — more than 60 — were nurses.

Many were charged with setting up a medical field hospital in Port-au-Prince, where by the end of the initial two-week rotation they had seen more than 500 patients, performed 66 surgical procedures, delivered 12 babies and had one death. Others worked with Project HOPE and the U.S. Navy aboard the USNS *Comfort*, a hospital ship anchored off the Haitian coast.

These were well-rehearsed responders. Among those first deployed were staff trained to work with the federal Disaster Medical Assistance Team (DMAT) and the U.S. government's International Medical-Surgical Response Team (IMSuRT), which is sponsored by MGH. IMSuRT's first-ever deployment was to Ground Zero following the 2001 terrorist attack on the Twin Towers in New York City. Members subsequently deployed to Guam and to the U.S. Gulf Coast following massive hurricanes. In 2004, after a 6.6 magnitude earthquake destroyed the city of Bam, Iran, the team was swiftly deployed, becoming the first official U.S. delegation to set foot in that country in nearly 25 years. The Department of Homeland Security honored the members of IMSuRT with its Under Secretary Award for outstanding work in emergency management.

Pictured at right, MGH staff nurse Nora Sheehan, RN, provided care aboard the USNS Comfort, *anchored off the coast of Haiti. Photograph by Astrid Riecken, courtesy of Project HOPE.*

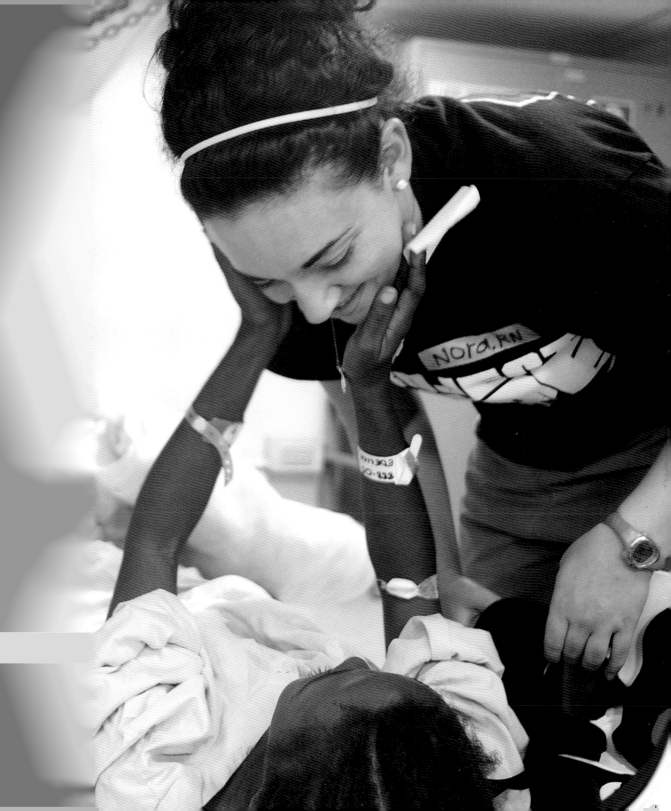

When the hospital's charter was signed in 1811, nursing did not exist as a profession, nor did the many other disciplines that today ensure the delivery of safe, reliable, quality patient care. We have seen phenomenal progress in 200 years. In 2011, as health care reform sits squarely at the forefront of the national agenda, health care itself continues experiencing rapid-fire growth and change. More than ever, the delivery of care relies upon an interdisciplinary approach, backed by a solid infrastructure of support and services. Leading the charge at MGH and within their respective fields are the members of the Patient Care Services Executive Committee.

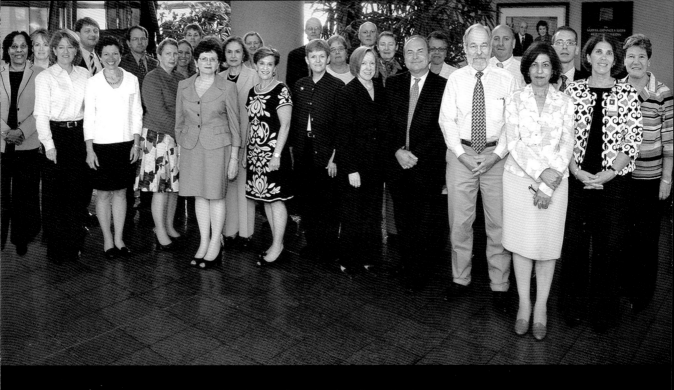

2011 Patient Care Services Executive Team

"When in distress, every man becomes our neighbor."

— *The MGH Founders*

As we revisit our history and look to the future, the many dedicated, compassionate and talented nurses of the Massachusetts General Hospital remain committed to preserving the legacy that is our mission:

Guided by the needs of our patients and their families, we aim to deliver the very best health care in a safe, compassionate environment; to advance that care through innovative research and education; and to improve the health and well-being of the diverse communities we serve.

MGH Nursing Leadership

Until the retirement of Ruth Sleeper in 1966, the director/superintendent of the School of Nursing also served as the director of the hospital's Nursing Service.

Nursing Education/Nursing Service

1873-1874	Mrs. Billings
1874	Mary von Olnhausen
1874-1877	Linda Richards
1877-1878	Anna Woolhampton
1879-1881	Jane E. Sangster
1881-1889	Maria B. Brown (1883)
1889-1909	Pauline L. Dolliver (1889)
1909-1910	Georgiana J. Sanders
1910-1920	Sara E. Parsons (1893)
1917-1920	Helen Wood (1909) *(Acting Director)*
1920-1946	Sally M. Johnson (1910)
1931-1932	Helen Wood (1910) *(Acting Director)*
1946-1966	Ruth Sleeper (1922)

ᘒ

Nursing Education

1966-1981	Natalie Petzold
1981-1983	Roselyn Elms (1959) *(Nursing Education moves to the MGH Institute of Health Professions)*
1983-1991	Elizabeth Grady
1991-1992	Judith Lewis *(Interim Director)*

Nursing Education *(cont.)*

1992-1996	Maureen Groer
1995-1996	Jean Leuner *(Interim Director)*
1996-2002	Arlene Lowenstein
2003-2009	Margery Chisholm *(2009, title changed to Dean)*
2010-	Laurie Lauzon-Clabo

Nursing Services

1966-1968	Edna S. Lepper *(Director)*

Department of Nursing

1968-1981	Mary Macdonald *(title changed to Chief Nurse)*
1982-1983	Gellestrina T. DiMaggio *(Acting Director)*
1984-1993	Yvonne L. Munn *(Associate General Director and Director of Nursing)*
1993-1994	Edward Coakley *(Acting Director)*

Nursing and Patient Care Services

1994-1996	Gail Kuhn Weisman *(title changed to Senior Vice President for Patient Care and Chief Nurse)*
1996-	Jeanette Ives Erickson

SOURCES

It should be noted that the following were drawn upon substantially in the writing of this history:

American Journal of Nursing

Interviews with current and retired MGH nursing staff

MGH Archives and Special Collections

MGH School of Nursing Archives

Parsons, Sara E. (1922). *History of the Massachusetts General Hospital Training School for Nurses*. Boston: Whitcomb & Barrows. Accessed via books.google.com

Perkins, Sylvia. (1975). *A Centennial Review: the Massachusetts General Hospital School of Nursing 1873-1973*. Boston: The School

The Quarterly Record of the Massachusetts General Hospital Nurses' Alumnae Association

p 2, 5. The circular letter appears in its entirety as a multi-page footnote in Bowditch, Nathaniel I. (1851; 2nd ed., with a continuation to 1872). *A History of the Massachusetts General Hospital*. Boston: Printed by J. Wilson & Son, p. 3-9. Accessed via books.google.com. Dr. Nathaniel I. Bowditch (1805-1861) wrote the first of MGH's histories.

p 11. Jackson, James. (1861). *Another Letter to a Young Physician: To Which are Appended Some other Medical Papers*. Boston: Ticknor and Fields, p. 129. Accessed via books.google.com. Dr. James Jackson (1777-1867), whose picture appears on page 2, wrote this book with Massachusetts physicians in mind.

p 12. Wyman, Rufus. (1822). Address to the Trustees of the Massachusetts General Hospital. The address is printed as Article VIII: Address to the Trustees of the Massachusetts General Hospital, to the Subscribers and to the Public, in *The Christian Disciple and Theological Review*. New Series: No. 20, March and April. Boston: Wells and Lilly, p. 129-139. Accessed via books.google.com. Dr. Rufus Wyman (1778-1842) was the first superintendent of McLean Hospital.

p 13. Nursing Conditions before the Training School. (1911). *The Quarterly Record* of the Massachusetts General Nurses' Alumnae Association. 1(2) p. 5-7. Accessed via books.google.com

p 14, 15. Putnam, James Jackson. (1906). *A Memoir of Dr. James Jackson: with Sketches of his Father ... and his Brothers ... and Some Account of their Ancestry*. Boston: Houghton, Mifflin, p. 162. Accessed via books.google.com. Dr. Oliver Wendell Holmes (1809-1894) made the quoted remark.

p 14. Jackson, James. *Another Letter to a Young Physician*, p. 122-129

p 17. Richards, Linda. (1915). Early Days in the First American Training School for Nurses. *American Journal of Nursing*. 16 (3), p 174-179. Accessed via books.google.com

p 23. Her passing was elaborated upon in the Trustees' Minutes of January 22, 1875. It was also recorded in Myers, Grace Whiting. (1929). *History of the Massachusetts General Hospital, June, 1872 to December, 1900*. Boston: Griffith-Stillings Press, p. 41, as well as the *Sixty-First Annual Report of the Trustees of the Massachusetts General Hospital, 1874*. (1875). Boston: James F. Cotter & Co., Printers, p. 15. This last title was accessed via books.google.com.

p 24-27. Extracts from the four-part series that Sturtevant wrote in 1895-1896 for *The Trained Nurse*, and which were later reprinted in other publications, appear in the chapter "Pre-Training School Days," in: Parsons, p. 3-18. Sturtevant, Georgia L. (1916). Hospital Life Before the Days of Training Schools. *The Trained Nurse and Hospital Review*. LVII (5), 255-260. Accessed via books.google.com

p 28-30. Much of the 19th Century Exemplar appeared in: The Writings of Miss Georgia Sturtevant, MGH's "Last Untrained Nurse." (2001). *Caring Headlines* Nov.15. p. 10, 12

p 34. Sarah Cabot Wheelwright Reminiscences [typescript]. (1904). Massachusetts Historical Society, Ms. N-173

p 34. Parsons, p. 32

p 36. Richards, Linda. (1911). *Reminiscences of Linda Richards: America's First Trained Nurse*. Boston: Whitcomb & Barrows, p. 26-31. Accessed via books.google.com

p 41. Richards, p. ix.

p 54. Scovil, Elizabeth Robinson. (Revised ed., 1894). *The Care of Children.* Philadelphia: Henry Altemus Co., p. 245. Accessed via books.google.com

p 64. Gruendemann, Barbara J., and Fernsebner, Billie. (1995). *Comprehensive Perioperative Nursing.* Sudbury, MA: Jones and Bartlett, p. 4

p 66. Perkins, p. 32

p 68. Perkins, Grace K. (1911). The Method of Administering, and Various Forms of Anaesthesia in Use, at the Massachusetts General Hospital. *The Quarterly Record of the Massachusetts General Hospital Nurses' Alumnae Association.* 1(2) p. 17-20. Accessed via books.google.com

p 77. Parsons, p. 160, quoting Dr. Richard C. Cabot

p 82. Parsons, Sara E. (1924). "The Nurses Point of View," in: *The History of U.S. Army Base Hospital No. 6 and its part in the American Expeditionary Forces, 1917-1918.* Boston: Massachusetts General Hospital, p. 57

p 86. We are grateful to Deborah A. Sampson, PhD, FNP-BC, APRN, assistant professor at William F. Connell School of Nursing at Boston College, for her personal communication.

p 88. Perkins, p. 49

p 90-91. This undated, unattributed newspaper photograph (reproduced) with article (not reproduced), from the family scrapbook of a 1919 MGH graduate, was accessed at www.deedy.com.

p 91. The text of the Van Dyke speech appears in several publications, including the newspaper article noted above, as well as in a news column, "In the Nursing World." (1919). *The Trained Nurse and Hospital Review.* LXII (3) p. 188. Accessed via books.google.com

p 102. Perkins, p. 301 describes the outstanding camaraderie among nurses and other staff in the Mallinckrodt Ward.

p 104. Perkins, p. 216, quoting Horner, Harlan H. (1934). *Nursing Education and Practice in New York State with Suggested Remedial Measures.* Albany: University of the State of New York Press, p. 10

p 111. Editorial Comment. (1906). Nurses' Uniforms Worn in the Street. *American Journal of Nursing.* VI (6), p. 353-354. Accessed via books.google.com

p 129. Weeks, Frederica. (1943). After Cocoanut Grove. *Atlantic Monthly.* 171 (March), p. 55-57

p 133. Perkins. This statement was accessed via books.google.com.

p 145. McLaughlin, Loretta. (1969). Nursing in Telediagnosis. *American Journal of Nursing.* 69 (5), p. 1006-1008. Retrieved from www.jstor.com Dr. Kenneth T. Bird, MGH staff physician, died in 1991.

p 149. Roberta (Goral) Nemeskal was interviewed for two front-page *Boston Herald* articles: Stephanie Schorow. (1993, November 10). Forgotten Heroes. *Boston Herald,* which contains her quoted remark, and Andrew Miga (1993, November 12). Healing Begins for Women of Vietnam. *Boston Herald.* Retrieved from proquest.umi.com

p 181. p 86. We are grateful to William R. Baker, Jr., Vincent Memorial Hospital, The Women's Care Division of Massachusetts General Hospital, for his personal communication.

p 202. Center for Nursing Advocacy statement, quoted in "American Academy of Nursing Announces 2006 Media Award Recipients" press release accessed at www.aannet.org

p 204. The first article in the series is Stefancyk, Amanda (2008). Transforming Care at Mass General. *American Journal of Nursing.* 108 (9), p. 71-72

p 219. *Congressional Record.* (2005). 151 (part 12) July 21, p.16837. Accessed via books.google.com

p 234. Bowditch, p. 3

If you are interested in contributing items or information that may pertain to the history of MGH Nursing or the MGH School of Nursing, you are invited to contact the MGH Department of Nursing at (617) 726-3100 or or the MGH Nurses' Alumnae Association at (617) 726-3144.

You may also visit:
www.massgeneral.org/pcs
or
www.mghsonalumnae.org

The MGH Department of Nursing

is pleased to acknowledge

the support of

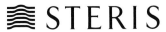 STERIS

in the making of this book.